ACTIVE ENERGY NOW

COMPLETE HYPNOTHERAPY PROGRAM FOR
EXERCISE & FITNESS MOTIVATION - INCLUDES 3
HRS OF AUDIO HYPNOSIS DOWNLOADS

RICK SMITH - HPD DHYP

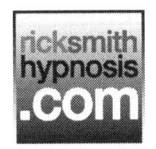

ricksmith
hypnosis
.com

The Copyright Bit...

This edition Copyright © 2018 by Rick Smith

All rights reserved.

No part of this book may be reproduced in any form or by any electronic or mechanical means, including information storage and retrieval systems, without written permission from the author, except for the use of brief quotations in a book review.

The Legal Bit...

I am a Certified Clinical Hypnotherapist. I am not a doctor or licensed medical practitioner, and I do not offer medical advice or diagnosis.

You're free to use hypnosis as you see fit, however if you have any doubts concerning it's efficacy in your case, you should seek guidance from a qualified medical practitioner.

Please do not play hypnosis recordings whilst driving or operating machinery.

Headphones or earbuds are recommended for privacy and effectiveness, when playing the hypnosis recordings.

CONTENTS

About the Author   v

1. Welcome to the Program   1
2. How This Works   11
3. The 'Active Energy Now' Approach   21
4. Using The Recordings   33
    SECTION 1 - HYPNOSIS TRAINING AND CONDITIONING   41
5. Why You Need This Training   42
6. Set-Up and Preparation   45
7. Stage One, Simple Induction and Emerge   53
8. Stage Two: Calibration - A Day At The Beach   60
9. The Training Transcripts   66
10. A Brief History of Hypnosis   80
    SECTION 2 - ACTIVE ENERGY NOW   87
11. Active Energy Now   88
12. Getting the Recordings   91
13. Session 1 - Take the Stairs   96
14. Session 2 - Choosing Your Future   103
15. Session 3 - Line of Commitment   105
16. The Transcripts   109
17. Program Debrief   144
18. Other Rick Smith Programs & Books   146

Afterword   159

ABOUT THE AUTHOR

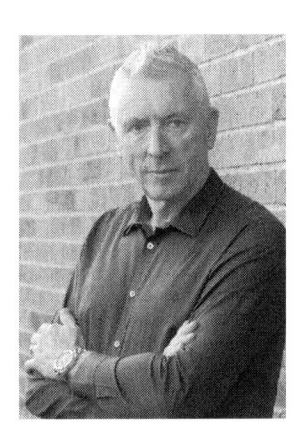

Rick Smith graduated as a Certified Clinical Hypnotherapist in London in 2006, and holds the NCH Hypnotherapist Practitioner Diploma from the Surrey Institute of Clinical Hypnotherapy.

His online practice, ricksmithhypnosis.com offers a variety of audio hypnosis programs covering areas such as Anxiety, Confidence, Workplace Stress, Procrastination, Weight Loss, and Health & Fitness.

Rick's book, *How to Master Self-Hypnosis in a Weekend,* has been a regular Amazon bestseller since it's publication in 2013.

Other Rick Smith Hypnosis Books & Programs in this series are available from Amazon or as audiobook versions from www.ricksmithhypnosis.com

- Cool, Calm, Confident You

- Do It Now - Crush Procrastination

- The Determination Diet

- Crush Anxiety Now

- Sleep Fast, Sleep Deep, Sleep Now

- Crush Stress Now

- Master Self-Hypnosis in a Weekend

- The Motivation Code

- An Ocean of Calm - Ultimate Tranquility

- Breaking The Ice - Social Anxiety & Shyness

- Sugar Free - Crush Your Sugar Addiction

- Stop Hating Your Job - Banish Workplace Stress

- Own The Stage - Presentation & Performance Confidence

Why not join me on Facebook...

https://www.facebook.com/ricksmithhypnosis/

1
WELCOME TO THE PROGRAM

SOUNDS EASY - SO WHY AREN'T YOU EXERCISING?

You know it isn't hard to do, but sometimes it's hard to start.

It's time to make a change.

• Maybe you're coming to exercise and fitness for the first time in your life.

• Perhaps you were an active teenager, but then real life got in the way, and you've not been trying much for a few years?

• Or are you a reluctant exerciser, already convinced of

the health benefits, but still struggling to motivate yourself from time to time?

Active Energy Now is my brand new exercise motivation hypnotherapy course. It includes three hours of original, professionally recorded hypnosis material, and it's ideal for anyone struggling to start or maintain an active, energetic lifestyle.

The skills and techniques you'll learn in these three full-length hypnosis sessions will equip you with everything you need; to start, maintain, and increase your activity levels, and prevent you slipping back.

It's all about ensuring that you do more tomorrow than you did today, and keeping that going for the rest of your life.

STAY ACTIVE - LIVE LONGER

Long-term inactivity increases the risk of arthritis, heart disease, obesity, stroke, diabetes, dementia, and an endless list of avoidable ailments and physical decline.

You have much more control than you think, over how long - and how well - you live. Whatever your age, being active will extend your life. More importantly, staying active ensures that you can enjoy your life, for longer.

It doesn't really matter what activity you choose to start with. Simply walking each day is enough for a lot of people to;

- rapidly improve your strength and stamina,

- enhance your circulation and lung function,

- and generally tighten up and tone your muscle system, which will be a huge asset as you age.

Once you accept and absorb the links between exercise, health, and longevity, you won't be able to understand how you lived this way for so long.

EASY CHANGES YOU'LL MAKE

Whatever activity you choose to do, you need a reason to start and a way to make it happen.

- In Session One, you'll be exploring the nature of activity in your daily life. You'll learn about making lots of small, simple changes in the way you move around each day, which will introduce regular exercise into your life *without you really noticing*. No running club, no gym membership, no sweat. Once you own this knowledge and perception, you'll find the motivation you need

to keep active, because it will simply become automatic for you.
- In Session Two, you'll explore the options for your future health. It's easy to put off thinking about middle age or retirement, if you're still young. But it's important for you to know that you have a choice about how you age, and you can make it any time. *You have control.*
- In Session Three, we'll examine and empower your commitment to your new behaviour, and provide you with the important tools you'll rely on in future, to keep you motivated, and protect you against slipping backwards. By changing your mindset in hypnosis, you'll change your real life.

And you'll feel a whole lot better than you do now!

You'll Succeed Faster With Hypnosis

As with all my hypnosis programs, this one will work many times better and faster if you're confident going in and out of hypnosis. If you've tried hypnosis or hypnotherapy in the past, and feel that it worked for you, you should be fine. If this is your first time, I recommend you complete my two short **training recordings** (included free in your download package) before you set to work on your new mission.

Hypnosis is progressive, and the more often you do it, the faster, smoother, and deeper it becomes. By conditioning yourself with the training trances, you'll find the therapeutic effects of the main recordings will be many times more successful.

Say Hello To The New, Active You

Once we deconstruct your present situation, and reprogram you with new ways of thinking and acting, you won't recognise the old you any more.

You'll feel powerful, you'll radiate positive energy, and you'll start each day with the all the active energy you need.

Each of the three recordings has a short introduction, or pre-amble, following which you'll begin the hypnosis. The three *Active Energy Now* recordings add up to more than two hours of professional hypnotherapy and training. All of this is easily achieved in the privacy of your own home.

All you have to do is relax!

THIS BOOK IS an extended version of my original audio download program. It includes:

- An overview of this program, the hypnosis methods we'll be using, and full instructions to prepare you for hypnosis
- My two-part thirty-minute hypnosis training and conditioning audio program, to get you used to going in and out of hypnosis, smoothly and easily. If you're already used to hypnosis, or you've completed any of my other programs, you can skim through this section, or skip it altogether.
- Three targeted hypnotherapy sessions to directly address the key components of your *exercise and fitness motivation*, totalling almost two hours of professionally recorded hypnotherapy.

You can download or stream the recorded sessions, free for life, by following the simple instructions in Chapter 4. If you'd prefer to record them for yourself, all the transcripts are included in this book.

Never play these recordings whilst driving or operating any kind of machinery. Please be responsible (I know you are).

How I Know This Works

There's a lot of snake-oil out there in the hypnosis industry, so why should you trust me?

Well, you already know that I'm certified (that's the big-shot letters after my name) so I'm ethically bound to provide my best professional efforts to my clients.

But if you need more: Here's a screenshot from my online store, which sells these programs in audio download format. As you can see, 42% of my sales are to returning customers (as of October 2018).

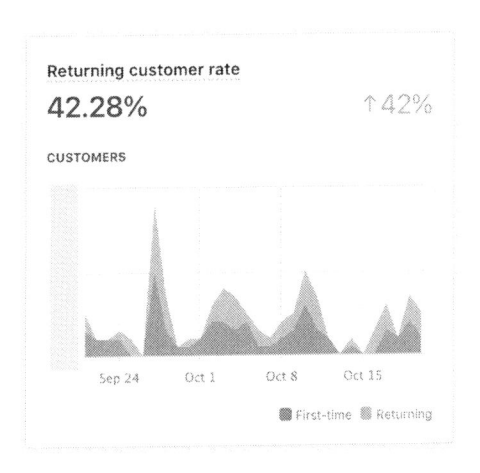

Returning customer rate
42.28% ↑42%

CUSTOMERS

Sep 24   Oct 1   Oct 8   Oct 15
First-time   Returning

So I guess it works!

Recordings vs. Face-to-Face Hypnotherapy

So, how does recorded hypnotherapy compare to a visit to the hypnotherapist's office?

Does this way work the same?

Well, it's not exactly the same, primarily because some conventional - *analytical* - hypnotherapy techniques require two-way communication between therapist and client, which is clearly impractical for us.

However, that doesn't mean it's less effective. Far from it!

Imagine this;

- You book an appointment with your nearest hypnotherapist, probably a few days in advance.
- For days you worry about the visit; *will it work, will I like the therapist, can I afford the cost, can I get time off?*
- The day arrives, and you're already anxious about the journey, apprehensive of meeting someone new, unhappy about the weather, and concerned about your work or family situation.
- You struggle downtown, with all the inconvenience and cost, and finally arrive, unsettled and stressed, for your session.
- You now put yourself in the hands of a complete

stranger, and spend the first half of the session wondering if it's working.
- By the time you're relaxed, it's over, and you have to battle your way back home, maybe more than a hundred pounds or dollars lighter.
- Once you get home, you try to replicate what the therapist taught you, but half of it's just a distant memory.

You may give up completely. Your problem wasn't solved.

The Alternative;

- You decide to try hypnotherapy to boost your exercise motivation.
- You buy, beg, borrow or steal a copy of *'Active Energy Now'* which will never be more than seven pounds / ten dollars.
- You find a quiet, comfortable space at home, put on your headphones, and listen to the sessions, which I've specifically created and adapted to work effectively in a *one-way* environment.
- You practice your new skills straight away, and repeat your hypnosis sessions whenever necessary, anytime, anywhere.

Now, how's that *not* going to work better?

Of course, there are many complex conditions which can't readily be adapted for audio hypnotherapy, and which really do benefit from the live clinical experience. That's why I don't publish programs about depression, addiction (except sugar addiction!) or grief.

Pretty much everything else works just fine!

∼

2
HOW THIS WORKS

How Does It Work?

FORMS OF HYPNOSIS have been a regular feature of ancient civilisations, some of whose rituals survive to this day. Shaman, Faith Healers, Cults and Religions have used and continue to use forms of hypnosis with their followers. Chanting, music and singing, sermonising, meditation, and even the use of psychoactive substances, natural and unnatural, are used to induce transient states in their followers.

Hypnotherapy is the practice of inducing this *trance state* in an individual (that's the *hypno* part) which suppresses your conscious critical faculty and enables carefully-crafted, congruent verbal communication to pass directly through the usual filters, to communicate with parts of the mind that are usually closed off to direct access - the subconscious - where habits and behaviours are stored and operated.

Everyday things like walking, talking, and eating are down there, as well as more complex skills that we acquire through our lives, like driving or tightrope walking!

Your subconscious mind is responsible for your automatic responses; how you act or behave in a specific situation. Such responses are learned over time, and sometimes, if some distorted information has been fed in - usually quite early in your life - your response to certain situations may be off-centre, causing you problems.

That's where the *therapy* part comes in. Whilst you're suspended in that open-minded, accepting state, the hypnotherapist will use his skills to change or adapt replace your habits and behaviour, over-writing your old, troublesome beliefs and responses with more appropriate new ones.

When hypnotised, you're able to accept these new 'machine instructions' unquestioningly, because the skilled therapist will demonstrate to you that your new way of doing things is more beneficial, and serves you better, than your old way.

As this is the primary directive of your automated subconscious – to protect you and ensure you thrive – it's readily accepted, and with application and repetition, your new habits are embedded for good.

The Stages

Hypnotherapy has several stages. Each one segues directly into the next, ensuring that the whole process is smooth and relaxed, with no bumps in the road.

1. Preamble

In the first stage, you're encouraged to find a comfortable position, and simply listen to an introduction. This preamble is intended to start the ball rolling, and focus you on the subject or issue you're going to be working on in hypnosis. Although this is not strictly part of the trance, it's a very important component of the process, and should ever be skipped.

2. Induction

At the appropriate moment, you'll be encouraged to close your eyes and begin the induction process. In this phase, the therapist uses a range of relaxation, visualisation, and imagination techniques to guide your descent to an adequate depth of trance for the work to begin.

There are many different forms of induction, some fast, some not so much.

In my courses, I start off using a specially modified medium-length and highly effective induction – the *Dave Elman Induction* – which is one of the most popular amongst experienced hypnotherapists.

In subsequent sessions, I introduce shorter, more rapid inductions, once you, the client, are conditioned to going easily into hypnosis.

3. The 'Work'

Once you are sufficiently deep in the hypnotic state, however that comes to you, the work can begin. Depending on the issue, there are a wide variety of 'therapeutic' approaches which can be used.

Here are just a few:

- *Visualisation*
- *Sensory Simulation*
- *Age Regression*
- *Time Compression*
- *Metaphor*
- *Coaching Techniques*
- *Breathing Techniques*
- *Re-Framing*
- *Triggers and Anchors*
- *Self-Hypnosis*
- *Pattern Interruption*
- *Modified Self-Talk*
- *Ego Strengthening*

For my programs, given the obvious limitation of tailoring the approach for each individual client, I have concentrated on using the optimum combination of techniques for these one-way recorded sessions.

We won't be delving into the dark corners of your life (if you have any) looking for eureka moments. You won't be beating your chest or clucking like a chicken either, I'm afraid.

You'll just be focusing on accepting that you need to make a change, and then making it happen, in the most appropriate, beneficial way.

4. The Emerge

Once the work is completed, you'll be gently guided back to a full waking state. You may remember everything, or you may remember nothing at all. As we said in the beginning, everyone experiences it differently, and I'm pleased to report there seems to be no correlation between 'reported' depth of trance and the effectiveness of the program.

5. The Debrief

After the Emerge phase, you'll be invited to review what happened, and the changes you have made. In many cases, I'll be setting you some homework, to practice what you've learned, and help to drive your new habits deeper so they stay strong and permanent.

This real-life work is equally as important as the hypnosis, because regular practice of your new way of doing things reinforces your new synapses, those connections in your brain which carry the messages between its different parts.

This is the science of neuroplasticity, the ability of the brain to rewire itself when required to do so. It works.

The State

So, now you understand how it works, how does it feel? And how will you know when you reach it?

It's practically impossible to describe the sensations of hypnosis to someone who's never experienced it, for two reasons.

- Firstly, because there are many, many different states, often unique to an individual. How someone relaxes and *lets go* is always coloured by their life, situation and environment. Everyone accepts hypnosis in their own unique way.
- Secondly, the state of hypnosis defies words, at least words of sufficient eloquence to describe it adequately. Can you describe how you felt in the last minute before you fell asleep last night?

You'll be familiar with that *in-between state between awake and asleep,* when your mind wanders and you start to dream, sometimes in short flashes, in between the little naps that drift in and out. So if you know how that feels, you'll be close to understanding how hypnosis feels – like hovering in that state, still aware, but otherwise detached from your physical environment.

But you won't have the words to describe it adequately, so there's no need to try.

Just accept it, and enjoy the experience.

Using The Scripts and Recordings

Each of the hypnosis scripts is printed long-hand in this book. If you want to, you can read and record the scripts yourself. Around one-in-fifty of my clients and readers appear to opt for that.

If you want a quicker fix - maybe you prefer not to listen to your own voice - I've recorded them for you, with my (professional hypnotherapist's) voice, and you can download or stream these recordings free of charge for life. The access instructions are in the Chapter 4.

It's easy, I promise.

I recommend you use your smartphone, mp3 player, or tablet computer as the quickest and most convenient method. You can carry the recordings with you, so you can use them anywhere, anytime. I've included instructions about how to do this on Apple and Android devices, and I'm sure if you're a Windows, Sony, or Blackberry user, you'll be able to adapt these instructions for your own device.

If you encounter any issues, please e-mail me at rick@ricksmithhypnosis.com and I'll fix it for you. A few of my Amazon reviewers have complained that they couldn't access the scripts in the past, and punished me with one or two stars. These issues are invariably down to a user's own settings, so if you mail me you'll get a quick solution, and I'll avoid any more negative reviews!

If you don't use a portable device, you can play the recordings from your PC or Mac. Somewhere in the world, somebody's probably listening to them on a cassette player or even an 8-track. Let me know if it's you!

You can download or stream the scripts by clicking the link at the beginning of the next chapter. You'll receive an immediate e-mail with your access details.

The System

Repetition is a key strategy with hypnosis of any kind, and you'll discover lots of opportunities to drop into trance and practice your skills.

Everything you need to know, and everything you need to do, is laid out in sequence. All you need to succeed is to follow the system.

If you enjoy the program and you find it useful, please take a moment to post a review on Amazon. When my first hypnosis audio/book - *How to Master Self-Hypnosis in a Weekend* - was published in 2013, there were maybe twenty books on the subject. Now there are hundreds, and most of them are disappointing, so if you find this book worthwhile, please help others to discover it by reviewing it. Thanks.

Now, just relax and enjoy the ride.

∼

3
THE 'ACTIVE ENERGY NOW' APPROACH

Introduction

AN AUDIO VERSION *of this section is included in your download package*

WELCOME TO THE PROGRAM.

Here's the truth about exercise: It sounds easy, but it's actually quite hard for most of us.

Even dedicated gym bunnies face their demons each morning. I've even worked with an Olympic sprinter who confessed to skipping training at least two days a week in the winter.

And it's so easy not to do it, isn't it. When that alarm goes off and you've got a choice between hitting snooze, or hauling yourself out to go jogging in the snow, your comfort zone usually wins out.

Luckily, these are extreme examples, and we're not training for a marathon - at least not yet - but the underlying psychology is the same for you and me.

Maybe you're coming to exercise and fitness for the first time in your life.

Perhaps you were an active teenager, but then real life got in the way, and you've not been trying much for a few years, maybe even a few decades?

Or are you a reluctant exerciser, already convinced of the health benefits, but still struggling to motivate yourself from time to time?

It's not important how you arrived here. By committing to this program, you've already crossed a line, and the skills and techniques you'll learn in these hypnosis sessions will equip you with everything you need to maintain and increase your momentum, and ensure that you don't slip back.

It doesn't matter how much you know about health and fitness: this isn't about the technicalities of what you do. It's all about ensuring that you do more tomorrow than you did today, and keeping that going for the rest of your life.

Now, this is not something I expect you to believe or take at face value. But please listen carefully, because this single piece of simple information, could easily change your life:

Quality exercise, done properly, induces a different state of being. Not only while you're actually doing it, but more importantly, when you adopt an active lifestyle.

Once you understand the importance of exercise and its ultimate relationship with health and longevity, then you'll get the picture, and you won't be able to understand how you lived this way for so long, without regular exercise.

Of course, everyone knows that when you exercise, you usually lose weight. Maybe this is important to you, maybe it isn't, but it's far from the only benefit.

It's really important to maintain muscle strength and mass as you get older, particularly around your joints. Life expectancy these days is more than double what it was three hundred years ago, so it's understandable that the parts of your body that move the most, wear out the fastest.

Well-maintained muscles provide support for these deteriorating joints, allowing us to stay active, and pain free, much longer in our lives.

Alongside muscle health, your circulatory system, which is your natural life-support, with your heart at it's core, needs to be maintained in good working condition. Regular exercise is far and away the best way to do this, much better and safer than drugs, and highly preferable to a double, triple or even quadruple by-pass surgery later on in life.

OK, so now I've scared you half to death – though I suspect you already know these risks – let me explain. It's a peculiarity of human nature that people tend to run away from things they hate, much more enthusiastically than they run towards things they like.

For this program to work, you need to enter with your eyes wide open. So it's simply common sense to make sure you fully appreciate what happens to people if they don't stay active. Their bodies wear out.

Now, on to the pleasure. I know, for some people it's hard to comprehend that there can be pleasure in exercise, especially if you haven't done it for years, but there is, and you may have experienced it before.

First of all, let's talk about altered states, and I'm not even talking about hypnosis yet!.

Humans actively seek out altered states. For some, it's alcohol, tobacco, or drugs. For others it's risk, like extreme sports or motor racing, because their altered state of choice is an adrenaline rush.

Many people have love in their lives, and that induces a euphoria that can be intoxicating. Foodies become ecstatic when they taste something new. Even the warm glow that comes with a chocolate bar and a Netflix movie is an altered state.

The commonality of all these altered states is that they all make changes to your brain chemistry.

Exercise, even light activity such as walking, can induce a powerful altered state. If you exercise long enough, there comes a point where you change from wishing it was over to wanting it to continue.

Precisely *when* that switch is thrown varies from person to person, and the intensity of the exercise. For me, it usually happens after about half an hour on the cross trainer. I have friends who run outside, and some of them get it within minutes.

For us, the important brain chemicals are endorphins. These little guys are the 'thrill' chemicals. You know how it feels, when you get some incredible good news, or you fall in love for the first (or even second time). Endorphins play a major role in sex, and are a strong feature in powerful leaders.

Endorphins also mimic morphine, with it's accompanying pain reduction effect.

The rise of endorphins, which your brain produces during exercise, is a short term benefit that's easy enough to achieve. When you feel it, you love it, and you want to do more, for longer.

The problem is that it's easily forgotten, and doesn't really cut it when compared to a lie down on the sofa with the TV on and a bucket of popcorn, when it's windy and raining outside.

But there's something more, something more pleasurable, and longer lasting. And that's what I call "The Burst". It's a feeling you get that's there all the time when your exercise starts to work.

Then, every hour of every day is accompanied by a holistic sensation: your physical body is bursting as the insides grow faster than the outside skin stretches to accommodate it. And the brain is bursting with the natural positive sensation that accompanies improved fitness and vitality.

Remember, you don't have to aspire to Olympian levels of fitness (trust me, I know some of these people, you probably won't make it). You just have to feel better than you did yesterday!

But if you don't try it, you'll never feel it, and you'll have a hole in your life, an undiscovered level of potential that would have been so easy to add, and which might just have bought you ten extra years.

If you smoke, you should quit. But it's not prerequisite. If you get into exercise, you'll actually WANT to quit in the end, because it will hold back your performance and the level of endorphins you can trigger.

Those sporty-looking people you see out on the street, particularly the runners? It would be easy to assume, from the generally pained expression most of them wear, that they are loathing every moment, every pounding footstep, as they strain to complete the run they've committed to.

You might think they're lonely, sad, and would probably prefer to be at home in the warm, with a cup of tea and a biscuit. It's a fair observation, based on the available evidence.

However, you'd be wrong in almost every case: nobody runs because they have to. They do it because they want to. Sure, some of them may not necessarily enjoy every moment. Exercise can be challenging, especially if you're just getting started or coming back after a long lay-off.

But the point is the outcome. The equation is very positively biased towards the rewards: the effort you put in comes back to you many times multiplied. No exercise is ever wasted.

And progress is swift: when you find a way to commit to a regular exercise schedule, you'll start to feel real benefits within the first week, and that will spur you on to upscale your commitment, as the rewards get better and the effort gets easier.

In this program, we're going to work on modifying your automatic behavior, in order to implant a more positive and beneficial mindset.

You don't only need a few good reasons to exercise; most people know what those are. It's more important that you have a reason to start, and a way to make it happen.

If you've not been taking exercise for an extended period, maybe because your job, family, or other commitments got in the way, the first step to getting in shape can be the most challenging. But, be assured, that once you've taken that first step, however modest it may be, the second step is half as hard, and so on.

The most important objective is this: if you do nothing,

you may not only die earlier than you need to, but also you may spend the final few years of your life in poor physical health, which you definitely won't enjoy, and neither will the people around you who may have to care for you.

Don't you owe it to them, as well as yourself, to be active for as long as you can be? You only get one life, so live it the best way you can, and stretch it out as long as you can.

It doesn't really matter what activity you choose to start with. Simply walking each day is enough for a lot of people to

- rapidly improve your strength and stamina,
- improve your circulation and lung function,
- and generally tighten up and tone your muscle system, which will be a huge asset as you age.

Your joints may ache, but if you surround them with good muscular strength, you'll stay mobile.

One essential part of your whole exercise regime is stretching.

The worst thing that can happen to you is that you pick up a muscle strain or worse, which halts your exercise routine, possibly for a long period.

For us normal citizens, not particularly pushing ourselves hard (unlike an athlete) most muscle injuries can be prevented by paying close attention to stretching.

If you aren't experienced, and particularly if you're over 35, running is not going to be right for you. It has huge potential for injury and is considered a *high-impact* activity. Many people's running injuries show up years later, when the constant buffeting of knees and ankles, previously concealed under strong muscle tone, finally takes its toll.

Try to avoid anything which puts shock through your joints. Swimming and cycling are better choices.

Whatever you choose, in the course of these sessions, make sure it's something that you can accommodate into your life.

My job is not to train you: I'm not qualified to do that.

My job is to get you out of bed and out of the house, so that regular exercise simply becomes a standard feature of your life, like eating and sleeping.

Because it really is that important.

Thanks for investing in this hypnosis program. I hope you find it useful.

As with all my courses and programs, this one will work many times better and faster if you're used to going in and out of hypnosis. If you've tried hypnosis or hypnotherapy in the past, and feel that it worked for you, you should be fine.

If this is your first time, I recommend you complete my two short 'training' recordings before you set to work on your exercise motivation. Hypnosis is progressive, and the more often you do it, the faster, smoother, and deeper it becomes. By conditioning yourself with the training trances, you'll find the therapeutic benefits of the main recordings will be many times more effective.

Training and Conditioning

As with all my courses and programs, this one will work better and faster if you're comfortable going in and out of trance. If you've tried hypnosis or hypnotherapy in the past, and feel that it worked for you, you should be fine.

If this is your first time, I recommend you complete my two short Training and Conditioning recordings before you set to work on your fitness motivation.

Hypnosis is progressive, and the more often you do it, the faster, smoother, and deeper it becomes. By conditioning yourself with the training sessions, you'll find the therapeutic value of the main recordings will be many times more effective.

The Training and Conditioning recordings come free in your download package, and the transcripts are printed long-hand in Section 1.

When you're ready to begin, make yourself comfortable and make sure you won't be disturbed. Draw the shades, eliminate any distracting noises, and prepare yourself to be hypnotised.

Each of the recordings has a short introduction, or preamble, following which you'll begin the hypnosis.

4
USING THE RECORDINGS

HERE'S how to access and use the recorded sessions, using your computer, smartphone or tablet.

The Hard Way - Record It for Yourself

In the next section, the scripts are printed long-hand. You can read and record them yourself, using your smartphone's Voice Memo or Voice Recorder function (or any other recording device), and then play them back as many times as you need.

If you're using your smartphone as the recording device, the easiest way to record your own voice is to use the microphone attached to your hands-free headphones. This avoids you having to hold the phone and gives you easier access to the controls. You'll be able to pause and re-start the recording as needed.

However, listening to your own voice is not ideal, and you probably don't have experience in reciting hypnosis scripts, which rely for their effectiveness on certain voice techniques.

So, although this is a perfectly practical way to work with the scripts in this book, I seriously recommend you use my pre-recorded versions as explained below. You'll get a better result and it will be much quicker to get started.

The Easy Way - Using My Recordings

All the scripts I used to create these recordings are included in the book. The Training Scripts are at the end of Section 1, and the Main Scripts are in Section 2.

Many clients buy my hypnotherapy programs as audiobooks from my website. The recordings you'll be accessing through this book are the same high-quality audio downloads, and you're free to download or stream them whenever you like.

How to Get the Recordings

The recordings are securely stored on Amazon Web Services (AWS) so that they can be played or downloaded 24/7. I chose AWS to host my recordings (more than 200, at last count) because of their platform's reliability and easy access for you, my client, on any device.

By the way, they're not paying me to say that!

If you experience any difficulties in accessing these recorded sessions, please e-mail me at **helpdesk@ricksmithhypnosis.com** and I will solve it for you.

My hypnosis recordings have been downloaded more than 30,000 times, and I receive one or two help-desk emails in an average week. I've simplified the access process so you should have no issues, but please get in touch if you do.

So, let's get you organised right now:

When you click on this link (or type it into your browser if you're reading the print version) it will open up a little form on your screen. Please enter your first name and your email address and submit the form.

That's all you need to do.

http://bit.ly/AMZEnergy

You should receive an email from **rick@ricksmithhypnosis.com** within a minute or two, containing your access information. Please keep this email safe, so you can access the sessions anytime.

It's not unknown for this first e-mail to go into your junk folder, so please check there first if you don't receive it within three minutes of registering.

In the email you receive, you will have two options. You can use either or both:

On Your Computer

The individual audio files are MP3's, the same as a song you might download from iTunes or Google Play.

Because the tracks are longer (30-60 minutes each), and there are several tracks in each program, they've been compressed and packaged into what's called a 'Zip' file, to make them easier and faster to deliver by download.

If you opt to download the .zip file, you will get the complete program (it may take a few minutes) on your computer's hard drive. From there, you click on it and it will open and unpack the individual recordings as MP3's.

Once you can see each of the individual tracks, you can simply play each one by clicking on it, or you can transfer the tracks (just like music) to your phone or tablet, using whatever method you would usually use for songs. If you're struggling with this, ask a nearby teenager to help you!

Alternately, use the links for streaming or downloading each individual mp3 recording. Using your computer's web browser, by copying or typing the link, the audio file will open (it may start to play). I recommend you pause the audio, then right-click on it, selecting *'Save Audio As'*. This should open a file saving dialogue box, and you can download and save the mp3 file in your music library.

Once you've done that, you can open your music player (such as iTunes) and find the track in the alphabetic list of all your stored music tracks. The artist name is Rick Smith.

If you download it to your 'Downloads' or 'Desktop', you can play the recordings direct, or open iTunes or your preferred music player, and import the file.

You can play it from there, or alternately you might decide to create a new Playlist (perhaps call it 'Hypnosis Sessions') and drag the track into it. Then you'll easily be able to find it, and when you sync to your phone or tablet next time, make sure you add the playlist and you'll be able to find it easily on your device, which is where you really need it to be.

On Your Phone or Tablet

Downloading the whole program's *zip* file to your phone or tablet isn't an option for most people, because these devices don't usually have a file system to open and store the tracks.

So instead, you can access the individual sessions and play (stream) them live, wherever you have Wi-Fi or data available.

Your *welcome and access email* will show you where to find the recordings, and it's one simple click to start, pause, or stop them at any time.

If you decide to go this way, you can be up and running on your portable device within three minutes of clicking or typing the link below, and you can always go back and download the whole program when you're near your computer.

This means you can access the recordings from anywhere you have data access. Each recorded session is typically 30-40MB (equivalent to 6 - 8 mp3 songs), so please be careful if you have a limited data plan with your phone carrier. Wi-fi, particularly at home, is often free or unlimited, so that's the best and most economical way to access the recordings.

Whenever you use your portable device for playing scripts - which you'll be doing a lot throughout this course - please use headphones or earbuds for privacy. This also helps to block out external noises, which can be a distraction during your hypnosis sessions.

All set? Good. Here's a reminder of the link that will get you rapid access to the recordings for this program.

http://bit.ly/AMZEnergy

And if you hit any snags, email me here:

helpdesk@ricksmithhypnosis.com

I'm not a corporation with a call centre. There's just me here, with a couple of dogs and the odd visitor. If you email during European daytime/evening, I'll fix it for you within an hour or two. If you're outside my time zone (for example North America, or Australia) it might take a little longer!

Now, go and get the recordings, and once you have them, we'll talk about the ideal set-up.

∼

SECTION 1 - HYPNOSIS TRAINING AND CONDITIONING

5
WHY YOU NEED THIS TRAINING

IF YOU'RE TRYING hypnosis for the first time, you'll benefit from some training and conditioning before we set to work on your Exercise and Fitness Motivation in Part Two.

If you're confident with hypnosis, and ready to get stuck in to the serious stuff, you can skip straight to Chapter 11 and start the main program.

However, even if you don't want to read this section, I'd still encourage you to play the two training recordings at least once, to refresh your skills and get you in the mood, so to speak.

You can complete the whole training program in an hour

or so, and doing so will greatly enhance the effects of the main recordings in Part 2.

If you've never tried hypnosis before, please do this training program. The recordings in Part 2 are *Intermediate* level and are designed to work best with clients who are well-conditioned in advance. These *Beginner* scripts will get you ready.

This initial training program contains two fifteen-minute recordings:

1. Training Session 1 - Basic Induction. This first session will allow you to experience hypnosis and trance, maybe for the first time in your life. You can repeat it as often as you like, and the more you use it, the more comfortable and confident you'll become with the whole hypnosis process.

You don't have to do anything except relax and enjoy the experience.

2. Training Session 2 - Visualisation and Calibration. In the second script, you'll explore your own capabilities whilst in hypnosis. You'll discover your *modality*; how you see, hear, and feel whilst hypnotised.

Once again, you may repeat this session several times, and your depth of trance and imagination skills will improve each time.

By the time you've completed these two sessions, you'll be ready to move on and get serious about your challenge.

~

6
SET-UP AND PREPARATION

IN ORDER TO give yourself the best opportunity for success with hypnosis, you need to pay attention to your immediate environment. The more ideal you can make the set-up, the more relaxed you will become, and the fewer distractions are likely to occur.

Most of these instructions are simple common sense, but you'd be surprised at how many people ignore the obvious!

Privacy

In the early stages, whilst you're learning the basics, you need to shut yourself away somewhere private, and make sure you won't be disturbed. There's nothing to be gained by having someone else listening in or involving themselves in the process.

If you live alone, it's simple. If you have family or flatmates, it's up to you if you decide to tell them what you are planning to do. In my view it's always better to come clean, because when you finally shut yourself away to practice, you really need to eliminate any concerns that you're doing something covert or sneaky, or that someone might think it's silly if they accidentally discover what you're doing.

You don't want to be trying to descend into trance whilst keeping one ear open for approaching footsteps!

If you're going to eliminate distraction - which is essential for this process to work - you must *control your environment*.

Tranquillity

Silence in your hypnosis environment is ideal, although it may be difficult to achieve, especially if you live in a city. Nevertheless you should strive to establish the quietest possible space for your hypnosis.

Close the doors and windows and switch your phone to 'Flight Mode' so that it won't ring or vibrate. Anything which disrupts your concentration whilst you're doing the exercise might take you back to the beginning. Once you're well-practiced at this, you'll be able to deal with external sounds as part of the trance, but at the beginning, until you've mastered the process, you need to eliminate as much external disturbance as possible.

You'll probably be using headphones, which will block most external noise, depending on the kind you use.

I regularly used headphones for my clients and a headset microphone for myself in my London practice, which was just 2000ft below the flight path for Heathrow airport!

Your Personal Comforts

As you've understood, achieving the hypnotic state will always go better if you eliminate distractions, which includes physical distractions.

- Wear clothing that doesn't pinch or constrict. You may want to remove your shoes, belt, and watch.
- Visit the the bathroom before you start. A call of nature half-way though your session is difficult to ignore, and it will probably mean starting the session all over again.
- Make sure the room temperature is comfortable; not too cool and not too warm.

Where to Sit

If you visit a professional hypnotherapist, you'll rarely see a couch or flat-bed in their office, and there's a good reason for this.

As you can imagine, taking people into a state of deep relaxation can run the risk of them falling asleep, especially if they arrive tired for the session. If you're lying down, the risk is increased, because this is most people's natural sleeping position.

If a client nods off during hypnosis, the session is essentially over, because your hearing shuts down as soon as you're asleep and nothing goes in, apart from the noise of a fire alarm or a wake-up call!

Falling asleep during hypnosis is not uncommon, and it's completely harmless. Once asleep, the hypnosis is muted, and anything that happens whilst you're asleep won't be effective.

Within the scope of the hypnosis exercises you'll do in this course, you can be sure that you'll eventually wake up 'out of trance', so no harm done. But you could waste time and effort, which is why you should try to avoid lying horizontally if possible.

Of course, if you have no alternative comfortable location, the hypnosis itself will work fine on a couch or bed, but you need to be aware of the heightened risk of snoozing through the best bit!

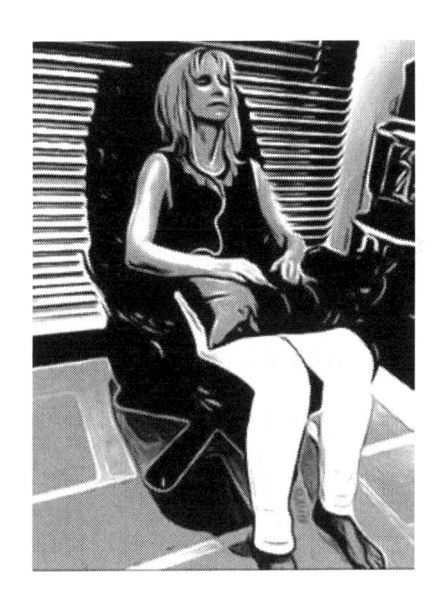

The ideal situation is a comfortable chair: even a recliner if you have access to one. Try to have your legs uncrossed and your feet flat on the floor. You should make sure your head and neck are supported with a cushion.

Where to put your hands is really related to how you would normally sit to relax. I've found that most clients like it if I give them cushion to put on their lap and then they can rest their hands on it.

A competent professional hypnotist can work on clients

in almost any position, and if you've ever seen a good stage hypnotist, you'll have seen subjects put into trance whilst standing up. This is genuine, but it takes special training and immense confidence to master.

For your purposes, you should try to get as close to the picture as you can manage. As long as you're comfortable, and you don't need to tense any muscles to maintain your position, this will work just fine.

Stimulants

Stimulants can be an issue, so you should avoid them. Coffee in particular can inhibit relaxation, so it's best to avoid drinking it before you're going to work on your hypnosis skills.

Later, once you've mastered dropping in and out of hypnosis at will, it won't make much difference. But in the early stages, you're trying to eliminate every possible obstacle to you being able to enjoy the relaxation state that leads to hypnotic trance.

If you're a smoker, especially if you're using hypnosis in order to help you quit, I recommend that you thoroughly cleanse your breath and hands before you start. In hypnosis, your senses can sometimes sharpen unexpectedly, and the smell of tobacco could become intrusive once all other distractions are suppressed or eliminated, which could trigger a craving.

Of course – and this probably goes without saying – alcohol and drugs don't go well with hypnosis. It's virtually impossible to hypnotise a drunk, and although I did once manage to put a hardcore stoner into a deep trance - after many attempts - the work we tried to do once he was hypnotised was completely ineffective!

Other drugs are mainly stimulants, and it's pointless to try.

Light and Dark

Given the choice I would always prefer to practice hypnosis in a dimmer room. You may have to open and close your eyes a number of times during the process, and if the room is bright this can tend to kick you out of trance more quickly.

How dark is really a matter of personal preference. During the day you should close your shades or blinds so that there is still natural light in the room, but no bright light source. If you're practicing in the evening, a side-lamp is better than a bright ceiling lamp. Try to make sure it's out of your line of sight.

That's just about it for your environment. Most of these

tips are obvious, but they all combine to create the most conducive situation for you to succeed at hypnosis, so try to consider each one in terms of its practicality for you.

So, you've got your recording ready, and you're seated and relaxed in a comfortable, private environment.

You're all set, so let's get on with the first exercise.

∽

7
STAGE ONE, SIMPLE INDUCTION AND EMERGE

What You'll Be Doing

IN THIS FIRST EXERCISE, we're going to use a standard hypnosis *induction* to start to get you used to how hypnosis works.

If you've visited a professional hypnotherapist in the past, it's possible that the induction part of your session may have been quite a prolonged affair. Many therapists use a technique called 'progressive relaxation' to take you gradually into a light trance, and then slowly deepen the state over anything up to an hour. This works fine for most people, but it takes a long time.

Rapid Induction

A famous American hypnotherapist, Dave Elman, having observed the apparent need to repeat this long-winded conditioning exercise, developed a very successful alternative which accelerates the induction process. I have been using this *Elman Induction* with clients for more than a decade, and found that it works well every time.

This induction compresses the repetitive conditioning into a series of brief *mini-inductions* which start to induce hypnosis through relaxation, then momentarily wake up the subject, before repeating the process again and again. The technique ensures that each time the subject opens his or her eyes, then drops back towards the trance state, they go deeper.

The result is a nicely hypnotised subject in a matter of a few short minutes. This is the technique we will be using in our first Training Exercise.

What To Expect

You won't be expected to make any earth-shattering discoveries at first, however each time you repeat this exercise you'll find that you'll become more confident and inquisitive.

Whilst you're in this light hypnotic state, you may find that you can begin to visualise scenes, places, or events. Alternately you may experience feelings or emotions, which can often become quite intense.

How you experience hypnosis will depend on you as an individual, whether you're principally visual, auditory or kinaesthetic by nature, or maybe a combination of any or all of these.

After an appropriate period of quiet time, my voice will gently emerge you from your hypnotic state, until you're wide awake, back in the room, and feeling great.

During Your Trance

Hypnosis is completely safe, and you will never lose your ability to wake yourself up if you feel uncomfortable with what's going on. The likelihood is that you'll wonder about this, sometime during your experience, but you'll feel so good that you won't feel the need to try to wake yourself up. I invite you to test this for yourself once you've gone through the induction stage.

There are three accepted stages of hypnotic trance which most professional hypnotherapists use. For the purpose of this explanation, we'll call them *light, medium, and deep*. In professional practice, the *deep* state is often used for treating really serious psychological conditions, as well as medical and dental anaesthesia.

It's unlikely (though possible) that you'll ever reach a state of deep (*comatose*) hypnotic trance using recorded hypnosis. Even if you do, the techniques contained in these scripts will work in exactly the same way, to emerge you back to your full waking state when it's time.

In this first exercise, we'll be targeting the *light* state. In this state, most people remain fully aware of where they are and what's going on around them, but they choose to 'switch off' that consciousness and 'go inside' to explore their own internal thoughts, images, and feelings.

You may achieve this light state on your very first attempt. You may even recognise it when it happens, or you may perhaps feel that nothing has changed, and you're just relaxing in a chair with your eyes closed. It doesn't matter, because each time you go into hypnosis you'll go deeper than the last time, and you'll discover new sensations and experiences which will encourage you to go further.

Remember, it's a *conditioning* process, and the more often you do it, the better you'll become.

When you emerge from your first hypnotic experience,

we're going to conduct a little de-brief, so that you can reflect on how you got on.

So, make yourself comfortable, put on your headphones, and when you're ready, **start the recording.**

∿

De-Brief

Welcome back!

How was that for you? Why don't you stretch now, I'm sure you feel like it. You completed the exercise really well.

Now, just take moment to reflect on what happened. You might remember everything, or you might remember nothing at all. It may have seemed like a really short time, or alternately you might feel like you've been gone for ages. I can tell you that the whole exercise took less than fifteen minutes.

When you're completely ready, you're going to start the recording again and repeat the experience, but this time you will easily go much deeper into hypnosis, and each time that you do this you will be able to go deeper still.

Right now, I suggest you get up and walk around for a few

minutes, maybe have a cup of tea or a glass of water. Remember, no coffee and preferably no smoking! Then when you're ready to try it again, come back and make yourself comfortable.

De-Briefing Yourself

After the first time you try the exercise, there may be things that you noticed which you can change in order to make it easier next time. Just run through the check-list below, and make any adjustments before the next repetition.

- *Temperature*: was I too warm or too cold?
- *Comfort*: how was my seating position, the position of my hands, and so on?
- *Volume*: was the recording too loud, too soft?
- *Brightness*: do I need to lighten or darken the room?
- *External sounds*: was I distracted? Do I need to stop anything, close any windows, and so on?

These are small things, but any one of them can detract from the overall experience, so it's really worth taking a little time to get everything right, so that there are no obstacles to you achieving that wonderful depth of relaxation which hypnosis offers.

You can go on repeating this exercise as many times as you like. You'll be the best judge how well it's working for you, and you'll notice the progressive conditioning as you try it again, and again.

Although my voice is guiding you, the actual hypnosis is coming from you. You're allowing it to happen, and it is happening. That's the essence of hypnosis.

You should not think about moving on until you're entirely comfortable with this first exercise. Many people report that the second time they do it, it's much more effective than the first, and this is the conditioning effect we discussed earlier. Just keep repeating the recording as many times as you like. There's no such thing as too much practice!

Next, in Stage Two, we're going to use the skills that you've developed in Stage One to train you to use the hypnotic state to do new things.

8

STAGE TWO: CALIBRATION - A DAY AT THE BEACH

Exercise Two

NOW WE'LL USE another recorded script which starts off with a similar induction to the one we used before.

Once you're in trance, you will be given a *trigger word*, which is 'BEACH' and your task is to experience everything associated with being at a beach.

The idea is to *calibrate* you so that you'll be able to tell if you're predominately *visual*, *auditory* or *kinaesthetic*, whether you see, hear, or feel more strongly in hypnosis. How you experience the beach will determine what we call your *modality*, and this will help you to anticipate and understand how to harness hypnosis' benefits in the future.

You'll be using your powerful imagination, which allows you to roam freely in hypnosis. If you're primarily visual, you may be able to generate a clear image of the beach scene and to be able to describe it, either during the trance or afterwards.

Maybe you'll be primarily auditory, in which case you may hear the sounds of the waves, or children playing in the sand.

Alternately - if you are primarily kinaesthetic - you might feel the breeze on your face, or smell the salty air.

It's entirely possible that you may experience more than one of these modalities, which is great, and it's also possible you'll form a multi-sensual impression, neither one thing or another, but which will work just as well.

This sessions called "Hypnosis Training Session 2" and you can download or stream it just the same as the first one.

Parts of the script may be familiar to you, which should help you to drop into hypnosis very easily. However, some of the parts are shortened because you simply don't need all the deepening techniques now that you've become proficient.

Again, if you insist on recording your own scripts, this one's printed long-hand in the next chapter.

Once you have the recording ready, make yourself comfortable and quickly run through the checklist below:

- Switch your phone to Flight Mode if you've downloaded the recording. If you're going to stream it (over wi-fi) select the setting which leaves the wi-fi on but turns calls and notifications off.
- Make sure you won't be disturbed for around fifteen minutes.
- Visit the bathroom if you need to.
- Take a few moments to acclimatise yourself to any sounds that you may hear during the exercise, and explain to yourself that these will not disturb you.

When you're completely ready, **start the recording** and enjoy the trance!

∼

De-Brief

If you followed the preparation instructions and stuck to the recorded script, you should be quite amazed by now, at your own ability to enter hypnosis and what you can do whilst you're there.

The Beach scene often evokes powerful imagery or sensations in people who try this exercise, and I'm sure you experienced something like that too. If, for some reason, it wasn't as vivid or literal as you'd hoped, don't worry. Just play it again, even two or three times, and the effect will increase as you get more proficient at exercising your powerful imagination.

You'll remember from the introduction that this was called a *calibration* exercise, and the idea was to try to discover your modality, that is to say are you predominately visual, auditory or kinaesthetic. Your experience at the beach should have given you a good idea of this.

Did you see the colours? Were they bright or dull? Did you see movement, or was it like a post-card? If any of these statements are true for you, make a mental note of the answers so that you can build your future visualisations around your strengths.

Maybe you didn't see much, but you heard the sounds. Could you hear the waves, the seagulls, the people talking and kids playing? Maybe you heard a more elaborate sound-track, like a beach bar or a restaurant with music. Again, try to recall what you were hearing and make a mental note of how vivid it was, how complex and/or realistic the experience.

Or maybe you mainly felt *things*, like breeze, smell, or texture? Maybe what you experienced was an 'impression' of the beach, enough to convince you that you were there, even though you couldn't see or hear very much? That's called kinaesthetic.

You should now be able to assess and decide your dominant *modality*. If you can't do it yet, I suggest you run the recording again, now that you know what to expect, and spend some more time at the beach!

You'll have accomplished this part of the mission when you're able to say to yourself: *"I am predominately visual/auditory/kinaesthetic."*

Remember, you don't have to have only ONE modality, but you should try to identify your dominant one, because that's the way that you'll approach your exercises when you start doing more interesting things with your hypnosis.

By now you should be dropping easily into trance, and you should be totally confident in your own ability. You can completely let go and enjoy the experience, and you should also have convinced yourself that each time you do it, you go deeper.

Once you feel comfortable with this process, you'll be ready to move on to the main event.

See you there.

∼

THE TRAINING TRANSCRIPTS

Session 1 Transcript

*W*HEN YOU'RE *ready to enter hypnosis, take a long deep breath and hold it for a few seconds. As you exhale this breath, allow your eyes to close and let go of the surface tension in your body. Just let your body relax as much as possible right now.*

Now, place your awareness on your eye muscles and relax the muscles around your eyes to the point they just won't work. When you're sure they're so relaxed that as long as you hold on to this relaxation they just won't work, hold on to that relaxation and test them to make sure <u>THEY WON'T WORK</u>.

Now, this relaxation you have in your eyes is the same quality of relaxation that I want you to have throughout your whole body. So, just let this quality of relaxation flow through your whole body from the top of your head to the tips of your toes.

Now, we can deepen this relaxation much more. In a moment, I'm going to have you open and close your eyes. When you close your eyes, that's your signal to let this feeling of relaxation become 10 times deeper. All you have to do is want it to happen and you can make it happen very easily. OK, now, open your eyes... now close your eyes and feel that relaxation flowing through your entire body, taking you much deeper. Use your wonderful imagination and imagine your whole body is covered and wrapped in a warm blanket of relaxation.

Now, we can deepen this relaxation much more. In a moment, I'm going to have you open and close your eyes one more time. Again, when you close your eyes, double the relaxation you now have. Make it become twice as deep. OK, now once more, open your eyes ... close your eyes and double your relaxation... Good. Let every muscle in your body become so relaxed that as long as you hold on to this quality of relaxation, every muscle of your body will not work.

In a moment, I'm going to have you open and close your eyes one more time. Again, when you close your eyes, double the relaxation you now have. Make it become twice as deep. OK, now once more open your eyes... close your eyes and double your relaxation... Good. Let every muscle in your body become so relaxed that as long as you hold on to this quality of relaxation every muscle of your body will not work.

Now, that's complete physical relaxation. I want you to know that there are two ways a person can relax. You can physically relax and you can relax mentally. You already proved that you can relax physically, now let me show you how to relax mentally.

In a moment, I'll ask you to begin slowly counting backwards, in your mind, from 100. Now, here's the secret to mental relaxation; with each number you say, you'll double your mental relaxation. With each number you say, let your mind become twice as relaxed. Now, if you do this, by the time you reach the number 97, or maybe even sooner, your mind will have become so relaxed, you will actually have relaxed all the rest of the numbers (that would have come after 97) right out of your mind. There just won't be any more numbers. Those numbers will leave, if you will them away. Now, start with the idea that you will make that happen and you can easily dispel them from your mind.

Now, in your mind say the first number, 100 and double your mental relaxation. Now the next number..... Good.... Now double that mental relaxation. Let those numbers already start to fade. Next number.....Double your mental relaxation. Start to make those numbers leave. They'll go if you will them away. Now, they'll be gone. Dispel them. Banish them. Make it happen, you can do it, Push them out. Make it happen! THEY ARE ALL GONE

That's fine. The mind is relaxed and the body's relaxed. Just let yourself relax much more with every single breath. And I do want your body to relax just a little bit more so let me help you do that. This time I will count from 5 down to 1. With every number I say, let your mind and body relax together like a team so that by the time I reach the count of one, mentally and physically you easily let yourself relax much more. All right?

5-deeper--that's good—4 - 3 --that's fine-2 – deeper down and ---------------- 1.

That's great, doing fine. I'd like you now to see if you would allow yourself, to let yourself, to go to your very basement of your ability to relax. And you know there is no real basement of a person's ability because we've never found a basement, only on every particular instant in time your basement can be many, many times deeper. And I'll help you to get there.

I want you to imagine that there are three more levels to take you to your basement of your relaxation.--levels -A, B, and C. To get to-level A,- you--simply- double the relaxation that you have now. To get to level B, you must double the relaxation you have in level A. And finally to get to your basement, you must at least double what you have in level B. To help you with this, I want you to use that powerful imagination of yours. And I want you to imagine that you're standing at the top of your own private escalator, like they have at the shopping centre only this is your own private escalator.

I am going to count to 3 - and at the count of 3, you'll step onto your escalator that will be taking you from where you are now down to level A, double the relaxation that you have now. When you get there, you'll let yourself know by simply raising one finger gently. Here we go-1-2-3. Step on to the escalator and go down, deeper down, doubling that relaxation which feels so good. When you reach the next level, step off your escalator and relax. Good, wonderful.

Now in a moment we're going to go from level A to level B. To get to level B, you simply have to double the relaxation that you're allowing in level A. Just let it grow twice as deep. All right. Imagine yourself at the top of your next escalator. Here we go, 1-2-3 and step on... Let it take you all the way down where you will have doubled your relaxation. Now, if you're following these instructions, you may find it difficult to move your finger, but that doesn't matter at all. But try anyway. Just take all the time you need to get to level B--- and when you arrive at the bottom of that escalator, step off and relax. Good.

Now there's one more level that I'd like you to go to: Level C -- the very basement of your ability to relax. Once more, find yourself at the top of that escalator. At the count of three, step on and it will take you all the way down to level C -- the very basement of your ability to relax today. Here we go: -1-2-3. - deeper-deeper-letting go-deeper-deeper-deeper-to the very basement of your relaxation-drifting down-much more relaxed. OK. That's fine. Way down. Now just let yourself stay there for a moment and notice at this level every breath you exhale just easily helps you relax even more. Every breath takes you deeper and deeper relaxed.

Now as you relax, drifting deeper with every word I speak, the first thing I would like you to know is how much I appreciate and admire you for the decision you have made to try hypnosis for yourself and to explore the wonderful benefits that it can add to your life.

Now you have those physical signs that allow you to know that you have moved from one conscious state to another in a calm and confident way. In this calm and confident state you can offer yourself generous portions of self confidence... large helpings of self-esteem, breathing out self-doubt as you relax even deeper and continue to enjoy the journey towards your goal.

Now you're going to take a short period of silence, relaxed in this beautiful hypnotic state, and experience whatever comes to you. See what you see, hear what you hear, feel what you feel, and simply let the waves of physical and mental relaxation wash over you.

(Pause)

You've done great.

In a moment, I'm going to count from ONE up to THREE. At the count of three your eyes are going to open, become fully alert, totally refreshed. Any cobwebs that you might have had, any sleepiness of mind is going to dissolve and disappear, and you're going to feel bright eyed and full of energy. You'll be fully alert and wonderful and marvellous in every way.

ONE, slowly easily and gently feel yourself coming back up to your full awareness.

At the count of TWO you're still relaxed and calm but notice that your eyes under your eyelids feel as if they're clearing, kind of like they're being bathed in a sparkling cool mountain stream, you feel GREAT.

On the next count those eyes are going to open, totally alert, fully refreshed, just feeling excited, wonderful, in every way, and every time you go into hypnosis you can let yourself go deeper than the time before because you know that just feels good.

All right, get ready, and on the count of THREE open those eyes and notice how good you feel.

∽

Session 2

Self-Calibration Transcript

When you are ready to enter trance once more, take a long deep breath and hold it for a few seconds. Now exhale this breath and allow your eyes to close and let go of the surface tension in your body. Just let your body relax as much as possible as you've done so many times before.

Now, place your awareness on your eye muscles and relax the muscles around your eyes to the point they just won't work. When you're sure they're so relaxed that as long as you hold on to this relaxation they just won't work, hold on to that relaxation and test them to make sure THEY JUST WON'T WORK.

Now, this relaxation you have in your eyes is the same quality of relaxation that I want you to have throughout your whole body. So, just let this quality of relaxation flow through your whole body from the top of your head to the tips of your toes.

Now, you know that can deepen this relaxation much more. In a moment, you're going to open and close your eyes. When you close your eyes, that's your signal to let this feeling of relaxation become 10 times deeper. You want it to happen and you have proved that you can make it happen very easily. OK, now, open your eyes... and close your eyes and feel that relaxation flowing through your entire body, taking you much deeper. Use your wonderful imagination and imagine your whole body is covered and wrapped in a warm blanket of relaxation.

Now, you can deepen this relaxation much more. In a moment, you're going to open and close your eyes one more time. Again, when you close your eyes, double the relaxation you now have. Make it become twice as deep. OK, now once more, open your eyes ... and close your eyes and double your relaxation. That feels SO good. Let every muscle in your body become so relaxed that as long as you hold on to this quality of relaxation, every muscle of your body will not work.

In a moment, you're going to open and close your eyes one more time. Again, when you close your eyes, double the relaxation you have now. Make it become twice as deep, as you did so many times before. OK, now once more open your eyes... and close your eyes and double your relaxation... excellent. Let every muscle in your body become so relaxed that as long as you hold on to this quality of relaxation every muscle in your body just will not work.

Now that you're totally physically relaxed. You are going to easily relax mentally. You already proved that you can relax physically, now you know exactly how to relax mentally.

In a moment, you'll to begin slowly counting backwards, in your mind, from 100. And with each number you say, you will double your mental relaxation. With each number that you say, let your mind become twice as relaxed. Start to count, and by the time you reach the number 97, or maybe even sooner, your mind will have become so relaxed, you will actually have relaxed all the rest of the numbers right out of your mind. There just won't be any more numbers. Those numbers will leave, if you make them go away. You have proved that you can make that happen and you can easily dispel them from your mind. Now, start counting backwards from 100 and make those numbers disappear. Each number that you say will double your mental relaxation. Start to make those numbers leave. They'll go if you will them away. Now, they'll be gone. Dispel them. Banish them. Make it happen, you can do it, Push them out. Make it happen! Good, THEY ARE ALL GONE

Well done. Your mind is relaxed and your body's relaxed. Just let yourself relax much more with every single breath. And I do want your body to relax just a little bit more so let me help you do that. This time I will count from 5 down to 1. With every number I say, let your mind and body relax together like a team so that by the time I reach the count of one, mentally and physically you easily let yourself relax much more. All right?

5-deeper--that's good—4 - 3 --that's fine-2 – deeper down and ---------------- 1.

That's great, doing fine. Now that you are so relaxed, you're going to go even deeper, and you already know how to do this. Imagine the escalators which will carry you down towards the basement of your ability to relax even deeper.

You know that there are three more levels to take you to your basement of your relaxation.--levels -A, B, and C. As you go deeper to each level double the relaxation that you have now. Use that powerful imagination of yours so that you're standing at the top of your private escalator and when I count to 3, Step on to your escalator and it will be taking you from where you are now down to level A, double the relaxation that you have now. When you get there, you'll signal by simply raising one finger gently. Here we go-1-2-3 and down you go, deeper into relaxation. Good, wonderful. (Pause)

Now in a moment we're going to go from level A to level B just like before. To get to level B, you simply have to double the relaxation that you're allowing in level A. Just let it grow twice as deep. All right. Imagine yourself at the top of your next escalator. Here we go, 1-2-3. And step on. Let it take you all the way down where you will have doubled your relaxation. Just take all the time you need to get to level B--- [WAIT]--Good.

Now there's one more level that you know you can go to: level C--the very basement of your ability to relax. Once more, find yourself at the top of that escalator. At the count of three, , it'll take you all the way down to level C -- the very basement of your ability to relax. Here we go-1-2-3. Step on... -deeper-deeper-letting go-deeper-deeper-deeper-to the very basement of your relaxation-drifting down-much more relaxed. OK. That's fine. Way down.

Now just let yourself stay there for a moment and notice at this level every breath you exhale just easily helps you relax even more. Every breath takes you deeper and deeper relaxed.

And now you know how amazing and easy it is to get to this deep place of relaxation, and you are welcome to remain in this beautiful place as long as you want and to come here again any time that you like, because you KNOW how to relax your body and mind completely and let go so you relax so completely.

Now you have those physical signs that allow you to know that you have moved from one conscious state to another in a calm and confident way. In this calm and confident state you can offer yourself generous portions of self confidence... large helpings of self-esteem, breathing out self-doubt as you relax even deeper and continue to enjoy the journey towards your goal.

Take a few moments to appreciate the peace and tranquillity in this deep place that you have brought yourself to. (Short Pause)

Now, imagine you are at the Beach and it's a lovely day.

(Pause) See what you see, hear what you hear, feel what you feel. Take a moment to experience how it is, there at the beach. Allow your powerful, wonderful imagination to transport you there and be at the beach, however that is for you.

If you can see where you are, say "I can see it", or if you can hear the sounds around you say "I can hear it" and if you can feel the warmth, the breeze, and the texture of the sand, say "I can feel it". Go on, just say out loud what is happening to you, and your imagination of this wonderful beach will grow stronger. Allow yourself to feel how good it is to be at the beach, how relaxed and comfortable you are and just rest there for a few moments, taking it all in.

(Pause)

And now you know new things, and that knowledge empowers you. You know about this beach, and how wonderfully relaxing it is to be here, and you know that you can return here any time you choose because you have proven the power of your wonderful imagination and your amazing ability to bring yourself to this wonderful state of deep relaxation any time that you choose, so easily. And I want you now to remember what happened to you at the beach today, what you saw and what you heard and what you felt, so that you can remind yourself later about this amazing beach and your clever ability to come here again. Just relax quietly for a few moments and take it all in.

(Silence for two minutes)

Now it's time for you to leave the beach for now, so let your imagination gently fade.

You've done great. PAUSE. In a moment I'm going to count from ONE up to THREE. At the count of three your eyes are going to open, become fully alert, totally refreshed. Any cobwebs that you might have had, any sleepiness of mind is going to dissolve and disappear, and you're going to feel bright eyed and full of energy.

You'll be fully alert and wonderful and marvellous in every way. ONE, slowly easily and gently feel yourself coming back up to your full awareness.

At the count of TWO you're still relaxed and calm but notice that your eyes under your eyelids feel as if they're clearing, kind of like they're being bathed in a sparkling cool mountain stream, you feel GREAT.

On the next count those eyes are going to open, totally alert, fully refreshed, just feeling excited, wonderful, in every way, and every time you go into hypnosis you can let yourself go deeper than the time before because you know that just feels good. All right, get ready, and on the count of THREE open those eyes and notice how good you feel.

∽

A BRIEF HISTORY OF HYPNOSIS

IF YOU'RE interested in how hypnosis and hypnotherapy evolved to where we are today, this short section might interest you.

If you'd rather get stuck in to the real stuff, you can skip this section; it won't make any difference to your experience with hypnosis.

What most people understand about hypnosis is largely grounded in two areas. On a personal level, you may have tried it, or know someone else who has tried it. Alternately, you'll have seen it on TV or at a theatre show.

The fundamental technique of hypnosis is 'congruent communication', particularly verbal communication. But the myriad of studies suggests that the process is much more complicated and sophisticated than that.

The urban legend that we only use 10% or 20% of our brains is an oversimplification, but it's entirely possible that we are only 20% competent in the use of *all* our brain faculties. This, of course, is the essence of training of any kind.

Hypnosis is a major part of the armoury of Witch Doctors and Shaman, as well as Faith Healers and Con Artists, who've been around since the dawn of time. It could be argued that the radicalisation of vulnerable young people by fundamentalist zealots owes a lot to hypnosis.

Some schools of thought believe that part of natural evolution is the understanding of the conscious ability to tap into the subconscious rhythmic operation of the brain and the body as a whole.

It seems likely that all the faculties required to enter a hypnotic state exist within a person's own mind, and that the role of the outside force such as the shaman or hypnotist is to guide the subject into accessing resources which are normally hidden, and to implant the skills to enable them to do it repetitively.

In the 18th century, a physician called Franz Mesmer identified the hypnotic state, and coined the term "animal magnetism", believing that it was an intangible fluid blessed with healing powers that was able to exert mutual influence between the Universe, the Earth and Animal Bodies, especially humans. He equated this fluid state as being magnetic in nature, and conducted many experiments using magnetism to demonstrate a natural or enhanced behaviour in humans and animals. In his most famous case, Mesmer treated a blind pianist and apparently restored her sight.

Unfortunately, given the political and religious environment of the day, Mesmer was labelled a fraud, and died in relative obscurity in Switzerland in 1815. However he left behind the term *mesmerised*.

Two notable British pioneers of hypnosis took the science forward in the 1800's. James Esdaile was a surgeon who used hypnotic anaesthesia successfully in hundreds of surgical operations, and in modern hypnosis the deepest state of trance is often still referred to as the *Esdaile State*.

James Braid, also a physician, was particularly struck by an exhibition of mesmerism by the French expert Lafontaine, and took up intensive research thereafter. During this time there was some confusion as to whether hypnosis was a state of sleep, and Braid's induction methods were based on eye fatigue. Braid's research has only become relevant and interesting in the 20th and 21st centuries, and he did not achieve much of a profile in his day.

After Braid, recorded research moved to France, and great strides were made in the use of hypnosis as a receptacle for suggestion techniques, and the language structures of *suggestion* started to develop. Sigmund Freud experimented with hypnosis for some time but eventually discarded it, probably because it did not offer him many advantages in his psychoanalytical work.

Fast-forward to the 1950s, and the era of Dave Elman. Elman was relatively low-key, but was widely regarded and respected in the medical and psychological communities in the USA. Elman may be credited with having taken away a lot of the mystique surrounding hypnosis.

Hypnotists of the day appear to have been somewhat anal in enhancing and dramatising the science and the therapies involved in it. There was also a great deal of fear around at the time, and the spectre of *electric shock therapy* in the mental health system frightened many people away from what they saw as *mental medicine.*

Elman dramatically simplified the definitions of hypnosis and also the techniques used to induce it. These days, confident hypnotists still employ the Elman induction, because it enables them to take most patients into a appropriate state of trance in between five and ten minutes, rather than the thirty minute inductions favoured by the more traditional branch of science.

I use the Elman induction (a lot) in my own hypnotherapy sessions, and it works well on almost everyone, saving a lot of time in the preamble stage and enabling more of the session to be devoted to actually solving the clients' issues.

Post flower-power, a new branch of hypnosis and psychoanalysis emerged, most notably under the leadership of Richard Bandler and John Grinder. The original concepts of *Neuro Linguistic Programming (NLP)* were laid out for the world in their breakthrough book "Frogs to Kings". Richard Bandler has gone on to have a colourful career but remains at the pinnacle of the NLP movement. His description of NLP as *waking hypnosis* may be viewed as something of a paradox, since modern science confirms that all hypnosis is conducted in a waking state.

Nevertheless, NLP aids the comprehension of language; how spoken conversation can be formatted to cut through someone's critical function and exert positive influence on the subconscious and instinctive part of the personality.

If you want to see a consummate NLP practitioner in action, I recommend watching one of Bill Clinton's big speeches, which can be found on YouTube. If you watch it, try to identify the small snippets of patterned language which may sound occasionally incongruous, but are carefully crafted to induce approval, compliance, or a favourable opinion from the audience.

Probably the best-known hypnotist in the UK, and subsequently in America, is Paul McKenna. McKenna makes hypnosis look easy, but he is without doubt an outstanding exponent of the science. McKenna is not just able to hypnotise people, but he has the sixth sense which allows him to quickly empathise with the subject, and thinking on his feet, use rapid techniques to effect a change. He's rich because he's good at this. I've spent some time training with both Richard Bandler and Paul McKenna, separately and together, and the experience was scintillating.

Many people credit Dave Elman with the quotation *"all hypnosis is self hypnosis."* The role of the hypnotist can be as a trainer. If you ever learned to ski, you can understand how it's possible to train a new skill into someone of any age from a zero start, usually in a matter of hours.

Hypnosis is a similar process: you have all the resources to enable you to do this, but you need a guide and a trainer to explain the system by which you access them and make them work.

SECTION 2 - ACTIVE ENERGY NOW

11
ACTIVE ENERGY NOW

Welcome (again) to the program.

My job is not to train you: I'm not qualified to do that.

My job is to get you out of bed and out of the house, so that regular exercise simply becomes a standard feature of your life, like eating and sleeping.

Because it really is that important.

Here's a reminder of what you can expect;

- In **Session One**, you'll be exploring the nature of activity in your daily life. You'll learn about making lots of small, simple changes in the way you move around each day, which will introduce regular exercise into your life without you really noticing. No running club, no gym membership, no sweat. Once you own this knowledge and perception, you'll find the motivation you need to keep active, because it will simply become automatic for you.

- In **Session Two**, you'll explore the options for your future health. It's easy to put off thinking about middle age or retirement, if you're still young. But it's important for you to know that you have a choice about how you age, and you can make it any time. You have control.
- In **Session Three**, we'll examine and empower your commitment to your new behaviour, and provide you with the important tools you'll rely on in future, to keep you motivated and protect you against slipping backwards.

Thanks for investing in this hypnosis program. I hope you find it useful.

If this is your first experience with hypnosis, or you haven't done it for a long time, please use my two Training Recordings which came with your download. They won't take long, but they will condition you to be comfortable going in and out of trance, and then the *Active Energy Now* sessions will work better and faster.

When you're ready to begin, make yourself comfortable

and make sure you won't be disturbed. Draw the shades, eliminate any distracting noises, and prepare yourself to be hypnotised. Each of the three recordings has a short introduction, or pre-amble, following which you'll begin the hypnosis.

Let's begin.

∼

12

GETTING THE RECORDINGS

Getting Your Recordings

IF YOU ALREADY HAVE THE recordings, you can jump straight to **Session 1**.

If you came straight here and missed out Section One (Training and Conditioning), here's a reminder of how to access and use the recorded hypnosis sessions for this program.

I've simplified the access process so you should have no issues, but please get in touch if you do.

Let's get you organised right now:

When you click on this link (or type it into your browser if you're reading the print version) it will open up a little form on your screen. Please enter your first name and your email address and submit the form. That's all you need to do.

http://bit.ly/AMZEnergy

You'll then receive an email from **rick@ricksmithhypnosis.com** within a minute or two, containing your access information. Please keep this email safe, so you can access the sessions anytime.

It's not unknown for this first e-mail to go into your junk folder, so please check there first if you don't receive it within three minutes of registering.

In the email you receive, you will have several options.

Quick Start

Just click on the Session link (1,2, or 3) in the email and it will start to play (provided you're online) on any device.

Download or Play on your Computer

The individual audio files are MP3's, the same as a song you might download from iTunes or Google Play.

Because the tracks are longer (30-45 minutes each), and there are several tracks in each program, they've been compressed and packaged into what's called a 'Zip' file, to make them easier and faster to deliver by download.

If you opt to download the .zip file, you will get the complete program (it may take a few minutes) on your computer's hard drive. From there, you click on it and it will open and unpack the individual recordings as MP3's.

Once you can see each of the individual tracks, you can simply play each one by clicking on it, or you can transfer the tracks (just like music) to your phone or tablet, using whatever method you would usually use for songs. If you're struggling with this, ask a nearby teenager to help you!

Alternately use the links for streaming or downloading each individual mp3 recording. Using your computer's web browser, by copying or typing the link, the audio file will open (it may start to play). I recommend you pause the audio, then right-click on it, selecting *'Save Audio As'*.

This should open a file saving dialogue box, and you can download and save the mp3 file in your music library. Once you've done that, you can open your music player (such as iTunes) and find the track in the alphabetic list of all your stored music tracks. The artist name is Rick Smith.

If you download it to your 'Downloads' or 'Desktop', you can then open iTunes or your preferred music player, and import the file from there.

You can play it from there, or alternately you might decide to create a new Playlist (perhaps call it 'Hypnosis Sessions') and drag the track into it. Then you'll easily be able to find it, and when you sync to your phone or tablet next time, make sure you add the playlist and you'll be able to find it easily on your device, which is where you really need it to be.

On Your Phone or Tablet

Downloading the whole program's *zip* file to your phone or tablet isn't an option for most people, because these devices don't usually have a file system to open and store the tracks.

Apple users are at a particular disadvantage here. I'm all Apple over here, and I haven't yet found an elegant way to do this on any of my devices.

So, instead you can access the individual sessions and play (stream) them live, wherever you have Wi-Fi or data available.

Your *welcome and access email* will show you where to find the recordings, and it's one simple click to start, pause, or stop them at any time.

If you decide to go this way, you can be up and running on your portable device within three minutes of clicking or typing the link below, and you can always go back and download the whole program when you're near your computer.

This means you can access recordings from anywhere you have data access. Each recorded session is typically 30-40MB (equivalent to 6 - 8 mp3 songs), so please be careful if you have a limited data plan with your phone carrier. Wi-fi, particularly at home, is often free or unlimited, so that's the best and most economical way to access the recordings.

Whenever you use your portable device for playing scripts - which you'll be doing a lot throughout this course - please use headphones or earbuds for privacy. This also helps to block out external noises, which can be a distraction during your hypnosis sessions.

All set? Good. Here's the link again that will get you rapid access to the recordings for this program.

http://bit.ly/AMZEnergy

And if you hit any snags, email me here:

helpdesk@ricksmithhypnosis.com

SESSION 1 - TAKE THE STAIRS

THIS INTRODUCTION IS ALSO INCLUDED in the audio download for Session 1.

Introduction to Session 1

Once again, welcome the program, and a big congratulations for making this new commitment to your fitness. Of course it's not really about the fitness and exercise itself, so much as the huge benefits your new strategy will deliver to your life, both in terms of longevity and also how active you can be, particularly as you grow older.

Please relax now, and listen to this short introduction to the first hypnosis session. You may close your eyes, or you may keep then open. Just be sure you're completely comfortable so that you can slip easily into hypnosis in a few moments.

If you're young, you might not be ready to think about how things will be for you in your sixties and seventies, but I will assume that you have an innate desire to live long and enjoy it. Our hospitals are full of senior citizens suffering from a variety of health problems, many of whom won't ever get better, no matter what medicine tries to do.

The vast majority of those hospital beds would be empty, if their current occupants had taken better care of their health and fitness earlier in life. Do you want to spend your final years doing that, or would you prefer to be active, engaged with life, and feeling strong and positive rather than worrying that every fall, stroke, or spasm might be your last?

If this sounds brutal, that's because life is brutal. But you can beat the odds; it's as simple as that. You are in control.

Of you're if you're already in middle age or older, your bad habits may be embedded deeper, and you may be daunted by the prospect of having to make big changes now, after a long period, or even a whole life of sedentary habits. And, I won't lie here; some if it might hurt at first, but it really isn't ever too late to start, or resume an active, exercise-centric lifestyle.

From the very first day you begin to work your body, even gently, all your key markers for heart problems, stroke risk, diabetes, dementia, obesity, and a whole range of life's natural born killers will begin to improve. Even if it's not possible to reverse the ageing process, it's certainly within your power to slow it down to a crawl.

And that's the point really. You'll probably work most of your active life, looking forward to your retirement when you don't have to work any more. You look forward to those golden years when you'll hopefully have time and the resources to really enjoy yourself, and do the things you never had time for before.

But more than half of us, and the percentage is growing each year, will reach our sixty-fifth birthday with at least one significant medical challenge, and in many cases this will be of such a nature as to prevent you for having that active, enjoyable, satisfying retirement. And the money you'd saved up over a lifetime so you could travel, or retire to the coast, will be sucked dry with medical and care bills.

Yes, that's the brutal truth. I can't sugar-coat it. Simply put, what you do from tomorrow forwards will determine how fit, active and healthy you'll be later in your life, when you need to be.

But here's the good news. There is absolutely nothing physically stopping you from exercising. Even if you have mobility issues, that leaves plenty of options for fitness conditioning using the parts of your body you can.

If you can't walk, lift weights, or row, or cycle. If you can't lift weights, walk. Get a dog, or borrow one. Join a club, a gym, or simply get out there on your own, whatever works for you. My job is not to tell you how to exercise, but to teach you to motivate yourself to do it, and eliminate excuses or supposed justifications for avoiding it.

This first session will inform you about things you may never have considered; easy small adjustments you can do to the way you go about a normal day, which will have a big overall effect and may, in turn, inspire you to greater exertions.

As they say, it's the little things.

Plus, we'll be exploring whatever it is we need to do in order to get you to naturally and automatically change some of the bad habits and behaviours, which currently stand between you and your potentially fitter, healthier future.

In hypnosis, these lessons will stick.

We'll go in slowly in order to achieve a satisfactory level

of working trance, so you can now allow yourself to relax completely, and simply listen to the sound of my voice.

PLAY THE SESSION 1 RECORDING NOW

Debrief

Welcome back! How as that for you? Why don't you have a stretch now, I'm sure you feel like one. You completed the exercise really well.

Now just take moment to reflect on what happened. You might remember everything, or you might remember nothing at all. It may have seemed like a really short time, or alternately you might feel like you've been gone for ages. I can tell you that the whole exercise took around forty-five minutes.

You may have experienced some strong feelings during the trance: that's intentional. You've learned already that your imagination is so powerful that it can cause feelings and emotions which are exactly the same, sometimes even more intense, than real-life feelings.

This is really useful in hypnosis because it allows you to sample how real things are going to feel, without having to actually take the risk of doing them. So you can test out the value of an experience in hypnosis, and then you know, as you do now, how good it feels to achieve difficult or challenging things, whereas before you might not even have tried them at all. You now know that it was your old, out of date habits and behaviours that were holding you back, and there's really nothing to be afraid of in everyday life.

Use this recording often. It's packed full of useful techniques that will build and multiply the more often you simulate them, and then practice them in real life.

Most of all – take the stairs. It's the fundamental root of the new habits and behaviours which will enable you to prove to yourself that even small, apparently insignificant changes to your attitude to your own activity can and will have a profound effect on your motivation.

It's happening in your mind. Your mind controls your body. So all you really have to do is think it, and you can make it happen, and reap the huge benefits in every part of your life.

Just because you decided to take the stairs!

Thanks for attending this session, and I look forward to working with you again in the next one, whenever you're ready to begin.

∼

SESSION 2 - CHOOSING YOUR FUTURE

THIS INTRODUCTION IS ALSO INCLUDED in the audio download for Session 2.

Session 2 Introduction

In the first recording in this series, you understood that you can find many, many opportunities to be more active in the course of your daily life.

You don't have to sweat in the gym if that's not for you; you simply need to be more active today than you were yesterday, and more active tomorrow than today.

We used the typical everyday example of taking the stairs instead of the elevator, but of course you already know that this is a metaphor for your whole life. Taking the stairs simply means taking the harder route whenever you can, and burning some energy by going that way.

This time, in session two, we're going to be examining different versions of your future, and you'll be able to choose how you want to be. This has nothing to do with your career, family, or anything else. It's about you, your body, and your life expectations.

By the way, if you want to use this recording in bed before you sleep, it has an open end and no debrief, which will allow you fall asleep without emerging from the hypnosis.

PLAY THE SESSION 2 RECORDING NOW

Debrief

As this session is intended for use in bed, there is no debrief section.

SESSION 3 - LINE OF COMMITMENT

THIS INTRODUCTION IS ALSO INCLUDED in the audio download for Session 3.

Session 3 Introduction

Before we begin session three, let's do a short review of the progress you've made so far. It's up to you if you close your eyes during this short preamble, however if you get yourself ready for hypnosis again, you can simply transition from the introduction to the induction without pausing.

In our first session, you took control of your options. Yo were introduced and encourage to 'take the stairs' instead of the elevator, whenever the opportunity arises. Now, you might have been saying 'But I never go anywhere where this is an option for me", but you know instinctively that this is a metaphor for how you conduct the active or passive part of your life.

Walk when you could drive or take the bus. Wash your own car, for a change. Clean your own windows, just don't fall off the ladder.

Any task that you can automate, just like taking the elevator, or getting someone else to do something that you, with a little effort and exertion, could do yourself.

You have now absorbed that motto "Take the Stairs" into your life, and you will always spot opportunities to do something small for yourself to use a little energy. It all adds up.

In Session Two, you were encouraged to explore your future, and that the life you can expect to enjoy is completely within your own control. If you do nothing, it will be tough. If you do as you have now done, and take the decision to maintain your exercise and activity levels as a major habit, you will definitely reap the benefits later on , when good health is more important to you than it has been in the past.

In this third session, we'll be equipping you with tools to help you commit to maintaining your active lifestyle.

With everything you now know, and everything you've now committed to, what you learn in session three will give you the permanent, automatic motivation to kick yourself into action when it's time.

This session is not suitable for use at bed time, because it has an emerge phase and a spoken debrief at the end.

PLAY THE SESSION 3 RECORDING NOW

Debrief

Welcome back! Time to stretch.

As you've learned in the past, everyone's experience of hypnosis is different. You may have gone very deep, and you may only remember bits of what just happened, or nothing at all. Alternately, you may remember everything.

It doesn't matter because the hard work is over for now, and you now have all the skills and resources you need to go forwards with your active, more energetic lifestyle. Your old habits and inertia served no purpose, and often held you back.

Use these recordings often, to remind you of the key tools and techniques that you now possess, and to maintain your motivation at the highest level so that it becomes firmly imprinted as a habit.

Exercise and physical activity is completely free, for everyone. You now know how to access it, enjoy it, and take the huge benefits.

I wish you all the best with your new, energetic approach to life's challenges, and maybe we'll meet again soon in a different trance.

For now, live long, stay active, and relax!.

THE TRANSCRIPTS

Session 1 Transcript

Induction

Now, take a long deep breath and hold it for a few seconds. As you exhale this breath, allow your eyes to close and let go of the surface tension in your body. Just let your body relax as much as possible right now, as you've done before. We will take it slowly so you can go deeper than the last time.

Now, place your awareness on your eye muscles and relax the muscles around your eyes to the point they just won't work. When you're sure they're so relaxed that as long as you hold on to this relaxation they just won't work, hold on to that relaxation and test them to make sure THEY JUST WON'T WORK.

Now, this relaxation you have in your eyes is the same quality of relaxation that I want you to have throughout your whole body. So, just let this quality of relaxation flow through your whole body from the top of your head to the tips of your toes. Now, we can deepen this relaxation much more. In a moment, I'm going to have you open and close your eyes. When you close your eyes, that's your signal to let this feeling of relaxation become 10 times deeper. All you have to do is want it to happen and you can make it happen very easily.

Ok, now, open your eyes... now close your eyes and feel that relaxation flowing through your entire body, taking you much deeper. Use your wonderful imagination and imagine your whole body is covered and wrapped in a warm blanket of relaxation.

Now, we can deepen this relaxation much more. In a moment, I'm going to have you open and close your eyes one more time. Again, when you close your eyes, double the relaxation you now have. Make it become twice as deep.

Ok, now once more, open your eyes ... close your eyes and double your relaxation.. . good. Let every muscle in your body become so relaxed that as long as you hold on to this quality of relaxation, every muscle of your body will not work.

In a moment, I'm going to have you open and close your eyes one more time. Again, when you close your eyes, double the relaxation you now have. Make it become twice as deep. Ok, now once more open your eyes... close your eyes and double your relaxation... good. Let every muscle in your body become so relaxed that as long as you hold on to this quality of relaxation every muscle of your body will not work.

Now, that's complete physical relaxation. And you already know that there are two ways a person can relax. You can physically relax and you can relax mentally. You already proved that you can relax physically, now let me remind you how to relax mentally.

In a moment, I'll ask you to begin slowly counting backwards, out loud, from 100. Now, you know the secret to mental relaxation; with each number you say, double your mental relaxation. With each number you say, let your mind become twice as relaxed. Now, if you do this, by the time you reach the number 98, or maybe even sooner, your mind will have become so relaxed, you will actually have relaxed all the rest of the numbers that would have come after 98 right out of your mind. There just won't be any more numbers.

Now, you have to do this, I can't do it for you. Those numbers will leave if you will them away. Now start with the idea that you will make that happen and you can easily dispel them from your mind. Now, say the first number, 100 and double your mental relaxation: Now double that mental relaxation. Let those numbers already start to fade. 99

Double your mental relaxation. Start to make those numbers leave. They'll go if you will them away. 98: Now, they'll be gone. Dispel them. Banish them. Make it happen, you can do it, Push them out. Make it happen! ARE THEY ALL GONE?

*That's fine. The mind is relaxed and the body's relaxed. Just let yourself relax much more with every general breath. And I do want your **body** to relax just a little bit more so let me help you do that. This time I will count from 10 down to 1. With every number I say, let your mind and body relax together like a team so that by the time I reach the count of one, mentally and physically you easily let yourself relax much more. All right?*

10-deeper-that's good-9-8-7 -6 - that's fine-5-4-3 2---------------- 1.

Now just let yourself stay there for a moment and notice at this level every breath you exhale just easily helps you relax even more. Every breath takes you deeper and deeper relaxed.

The Work

As you now embark on this journey, we should take a moment mark your achievements, which have already begun with you taking the first steps. You have decided to make changes, and these changes you have decided to make will alter and enhance your life from this day forwards.

And the phrase 'this day forwards' is more important to you today than before, and more important to you than it is to other people, because on this day, the changes you make will be creating a new version of you; a, stronger, happier version who puts a high priority on improving your health and vitality every minute of every hour of every day.

Because you already know that's how health works. Although there are some people, about who you may heard it said, they have good genes, and natural health, you also instinctively know, that even these people, take daily, active steps, to maintain and improve their fitness, because being like those people just feels good, much better that you may be feeling now.

And you might be curious, as you descend more deeply, if it is possible for you to be like that, to join that group of healthy looking, healthy feeling people. So I have some good news for you. You can become like that, and you have all the personal resources you'll need to get there. And it won't take very long at all, once you accept the truth that you only have to think a little differently, and you only have to act a little differently, for it to become true for you.

All you have to do is to want it to happen, and you will make it happen.

In a moment, I'd like to invite you to use your powerful imagination.

As you relax deeper and listen to the sound of my voice, I'd like you to imagine you're standing in the entrance foyer of a building in the city or town near you. Perhaps this building is somewhere you've been before, or maybe it's a building you've seen on TV or in a movie. Take a moment to be in that place.

Good.

From where you're standing, you're facing a bank of elevators, and you watch the little red numbers above the elevator doors as they rise and fall from floor to floor, carrying people from one level to another, up and down, never pausing for longer than a few seconds to let people in or out. As you watch, each of the elevators in turn arrives at the ground floor, and the doors swish open. All those people walk out of the elevator and disperse in different directions, and new people get into the empty elevators, the doors swish closed, and you watch as those little red numbers start to change again.

Now, you're here in this building for a reason; you have to deliver an package to someone in one of the offices. You don't know what is in the package, because you're doing a favour for a friend, and that doesn't matter right now.

You look at the address label on the package and you see that the office you want is on the third floor of this building, even though there are many more floors. All you have to do is to go up to the third floor, hand the package to the receptionist, and come down again.

From where you are now, you can easily notice that there is a staircase alongside the elevators. Some of the people who come into the building head straight for the elevator, and some people head for the stairs. You begin to notice that those people who are using the elevators are different from those people who take the stairs.

The people who take the stairs move more quickly, and appear more active. The people who take the stairs have no need to wait around for an elevator to arrive, because there's never a queue for the stairs, so they arrive, take the stairs, and move on to the next place.

The people who take the stairs are positive. They know they are going to take the stairs before they even enter the building, because it is their habit to take the stairs whenever the option to take the stairs exists.

Now you're thinking that you would perhaps like to try taking the stairs, but you usually take the elevator, and you're anxious to deliver your package to the third floor, so you step closer to the elevators, and when one of the cars arrives, you join the crush and squeeze inside.

The elevator fills up quickly with people. You notice that it's quite hot inside, and you're crushed in a corner by the weight of people. The doors swish closed and you feel the car begin to move, slowly, but you know you're rising up, heading for the first floor.

This elevator is so slow. You can see the numbers above the door, and for an interminable time it flashes zero, for the ground floor, until eventually the number One appears, but still the car moves slowly, and the heat and stuffiness inside grows more uncomfortable.

Then the elevator stops and, after a pause, the doors swish slowly open. A few people leave at the first floor, but even more people cram in to the already overcrowded car. Maybe you're feeling impatient now, because this elevator is so slow, and it's so hot and crowded inside. You are beginning too wish that you'd taken the stairs.

Finally, the doors slide closed and the car begins to move again, very slowly, heading upwards to the second floor. You continue to watch and observe the numbers above the door, and after a little while the number one changes to the number two, as you approach the second floor.

And now, you begin to sense something important. You start to realise that every number that appears above the elevator door is not only the number for the next floor where the car will stop. This elevator is different to any other elevator you've travelled in before. This elevator is counting for <u>you</u>.

The numbers are not only the floors, but as they ascend, going from zero, to one, and now from one to two, you understand that these numbers are actually counting minutes. Not minutes that are happening now, but minutes that can be subtracted from the end of your life. Each floor you ascend in this elevator costs you one minute of life.

The longer you spend in that elevator, the more minutes you are wasting, minute that may not seem valuable to you now, because these minutes will be taken from you long in the future. When you need those minutes, they will be the most precious minutes of your life, but you will have to give them up, because you took the elevator.

Now you understand the cost in minutes of riding the elevator, and the car slows once again as it approaches the second floor. You know that you've already spent two minutes from the end of your life.

And now you have this knowledge, and you understand that riding the elevator is hot, cramped, smelly, and now it is costing you time which you'll lose from your life in the future, you find that you are confident to take a new decision about how you invest, spend, and receive time in your life.

Perhaps it's time you stopped that time from slipping away. Perhaps its time to get out of that elevator before you lose any more minutes, because minutes become hours, and hours become days

But you only have one more floor to go, so you need to decide if you are prepared to sacrifice one more minute in order to save the effort, because you briefly recall that the active healthy looking people you saw earlier will have taken the stairs, and you instinctively know that if you take the stairs you will immediately stop these valuable minutes from slipping away, because when you give away your minutes like this, simply because you haven't yet decided to invest the effort to keep these minutes for when you will need them, there is no positive benefit, you are simply burning precious time when there is a better way.

And now the elevator slows to a gentle stop at the second floor, and you have made a decision, a decision that you automatically know is going to be of huge benefit to you, now and in the future, so you push your way through the crowd and step out of the elevator.

As you make your way through to the door, you can instinctively feel, see and hear that the people in the elevator haven't yet realised how the numbers work, and that the are giving away minutes from their own lives, simply by staying in the elevator, but you know better, and you can use that knowledge properly, and indeed you need never give away your time again, for such a pointless reason.

You'll try taking the stairs. It's only one more floor, and you can go at your own speed.

You step out of the elevator, and take the first step on the stair-

case, then the second. You feel the extra effort and exertion, first in your legs, because you can't remember a time before, when you would take the stairs as a preference to an easy ride up in an elevator.

And as you climb the stairs, not too fast and not to slow, you begin to understand that these stairs are also special, just like the elevator that was counting away those precious minutes of life, these stairs work in reverse.

Instead of spending your minutes in the elevator, shortening your life, this staircase rewards your effort, as for every step you climb, you are awarded an free minute, added to the end of your life. Every step you climb adds one more minute, precious time that you'll be able to use to extend your life.

And as you climb these stairs, you count the minutes that are being added to your life

One step gives you one minute

The second step gives you a second minute

The third step means you've now added three bonus minutes.

And each step you take adds one more minute to your life.

As you gently climb these stairs, you can notice that your legs are perhaps growing a little tired, and your heart begins to beat a little faster, and your breathing increases, but you don't need to worry about it now because you know that its perfectly normal, and in the future the more often you take the stairs, the easier it will become for you, and you'll start to look for opportunities to take the stairs every time, in preference to making no effort by taking the elevator and giving away all those valuable minutes, now you know that you can earn minutes and add them to your lifespan, and it's a simple as taking the stairs.

And from today forwards, you know instinctively that this change has happened, and that you will always prefer to take the stairs, any time you get the opportunity, and to add more bonus free minutes to your life, and you know that this is an almost unlimited reserve of time which belongs to you, and all you have to do is reclaim it, by taking the stairs.

Because you are now that person that prefers to make a small physical effort, whenever the opportunity arises, to add a few extra minutes, and you'll no longer accept giving away valuable time by taking the easy way, or the lazy way.

From this day forwards you'll be constantly alert, looking for opportunities to earn time, and not spend it. By taking the stairs instead of the elevator, you'll add minutes.

By walking to the shop instead of driving, you'll add minutes.

By going outside and walking around, instead of staying inside on the sofa, you'll add minutes.

And all these small adjustments that you're now making,

because you have understood how easy and simple it is to earn those extra minutes, and as you make these new habits and behaviours a regular feature in your life, soon those minutes will add up to hours, then to days and weeks, and soon you find that your new, active approach to each and every day adds up to years of additional, active, healthy life.

All because you decided to take the stairs.

In your imagination you may form an impression of your old self, perhaps when you used to take the elevator; see what you see, hear what you hear, and feel what you feel. And when that impression of your old self is clearer, let it fade, let it shrink, let it recede into the distance. You don't need that impression of your old self any more. You have proved that you have all the resources you need to make the changes you desire.

You have a new way to be. You are changing, because you've decided to change. You are that person that takes the stairs.

You may continue to imagine all the ways, in which your new behaviour will now benefit you, and those around you, or you may decide to switch off your thoughts, and just enjoy this time of peace and solitude. So just take a moment of quietness at your leisure, starting now...

<<pause>>

Very good. Thank you for your focus and co-operation, you've been excellent in every way.

You've done great.

Emerge

PAUSE. In a moment I'm going to count from ONE up to THREE. At the count of three your eyes are going to open, become fully alert, totally refreshed. Any cobwebs that you might have had, any sleepiness of mind is going to dissolve and disappear, and you're going to feel bright eyed and full of energy.

You'll be fully alert and wonderful and marvellous in every way.

ONE, slowly easily and gently feel yourself coming back up to your full awareness,

At the count of TWO you're still relaxed and calm but notice that your eyes under your eyelids feel as if they're clearing, kind of like they're being bathed in a sparkling cool mountain stream, you feel GREAT.

On the next count those eyes are going to open, totally alert, fully refreshed, just feeling excited, wonderful, in every way, and every time you go into hypnosis you can let yourself go deeper than the time before because you know that just feels good.

All right, get ready, and on the count of THREE open those eyes and notice how good you feel.

Session 2 Transcript

Induction

So, once you've settled yourself, close your eyes, and let's start by taking the deep breath in, as usual, and this time, as you breathe out to start the journey, just allow yourself to smile a little, so that the descent into trance will be even more pleasurable than usual.

And breathe in – smile – breathe out, and feel a warm wave of relaxation spreading throughout your whole body, loosening and relaxing all the muscles around your joints, and just allowing yourself to push out any residual tension from those muscles and joints, just allowing yourself to go limp and floppy, lazy and relaxed, as you drift downwards into that calm, relaxed state where you have already demonstrated that you can make excellent and marvellous changes.

Now, you have often shown in the past that you are highly receptive to hypnosis, and that you can now go deeper and quicker into trance than the majority of people. So you know that even now you are already much deeper than when you first started enjoying hypnosis because you have had so many interesting and remarkable experiences, and the things that you learned and discovered have already begun to benefit your life, so you can fully allow yourself to go deeper still, while you listen to the sound of my voice.

As you drift deeper down now, noticing the regularity of your breathing, and how the effect of breathing out each time leads you down deeper, more relaxed, and already you may be curious about what it is that you will learn this time, because every time you come here you learn new things, and every time your repeat those things you learn, they empower and support you more each day,

And you might wonder if there is any limit to the things you can learn or the habits you can change when you are in this relaxed, deep, comfortable, safe space, and I can tell you that there are no limits, because no-one has discovered the limits, as no-one has found any limit to how deeply relaxed you can become, so you can always go deeper, and you will go deeper now, so go on – let yourself go deeper now.

That's good, you're now so deep that you know that your body is completely relaxed, and your mind is open and ready to receive new learning, that you can add new resources that will strengthen you.

And I want you to know that everything we're going to do today is scientific. Everything we do today will use the power of knowledge to affect the parts of you, the parts of your body itself, that determine how you respond, in every situation. And you already learned how to do this, and now you're going to learn how to make yourself more powerful, stronger, and more resilient.

Now, as you drift gently downwards into a deeper state of relaxation, conscious only of the gently rhythm of your breathing and the sound of my voice, I have some more useful information that you might like to know

THE WORK

Before today, it may have been your experience that it was difficult to find either the time or the energy to exercise regularly. You have always known that more activity would be of great benefit to your life, and you may have had periods in your life where you were more active than now, so you already understand when you stay active, you feel good all the time.

And you might be curious to understand why you have, until today, allowed and permitted thoughts and feelings to overrule your clear knowledge that being active is good for you.

And in this deepened, relaxed state of consciousness, you can now acknowledge that it's a good time for you to make a change.

Human beings - and other animals too - were designed to move - in primitive times we were very lean and fit and sprightly - we had to move fast when we were faced with danger - had to compete with our fellow humans - for survival - it was an inborn instinct.

Nature has created humans and animals with the capability to move around, as a necessary part of your survival. Sometimes we move around slowly, looking and browsing the world as we see it. And sometimes we can move faster, when we are in a hurry, or we are in danger or facing a threat. Our bodies have evolved with both these capabilities, to move slowly and conserve our physical energy, always ready to move fast if we need to or if we want to.

For some people, they lose their balance and spend more time in the slow, energy conservation zone. They take false comfort from relaxation, as do we all, however they can sometimes forget the pleasure that can be taken from more energetic movement, which balances their lives with health and vitality..

For many people, if this imbalance is permitted for long enough, as they near old age, they will begin to notice their physical movement becoming more challenging, and even restricted. At this time of life, which we must all inevitably face, you may regret that it could have been so easy to made different choices, and pursued a different balance, a more active lifestyle.

It doesn't have to be like that though - because for any change in your life - a change must first take place in your mind - and you can change your mind whenever you wish - and you're here right now because it is your wish - your desire - to begin to really enjoy being more active.

And all you have to do is to want it to happen, and you will make it happen.

Maybe there was a time earlier when you enjoyed exercise, and you understand the pleasure chemicals that flood your brain when you exercise correctly, which is the best and most enjoyable part of activity. The rush of exercise can easily become a positive addiction; the more you get, the more you want, and that desire can support and motivate you to exercise more often.

Now, I'm going to ask you to call on your powerful imagination, as you've done before.

I'd like you to use your powers of imagination and visualisation, to imagine yourself now, standing still in the warm sunshine, out in the country. You're standing in the middle of a deserted road, and you are aware that you've traveled some distance to arrive here.

The road behind you represents your life, and the years that have passed on your journey to this calm, pleasant place. The road ahead represents your future, and all the things that you'll experience from now onwards.

Be there, standing in the road, see what you see, hear what you hear, feel what you feel.

Ahead of you, you can see that the road divides in two, at a fork. You begin to walk slowly along the road, now going down a gentle incline, until you reach the fork in the road. Allow yourself to stop there for a moment and rest.

As you look down the road on the left you, understand that this road represents your life for the next few years if you choose to continue down your present path, the path of allowing outside influences to obstruct you from being physically active, just for a short time each day.

Because you're curious and you always believe in having all the information you need to support your decision to change, you find yourself drawn to explore this road for a while, always knowing that you can come back to the fork any time you like.

You begin to walk, and as you travel slowly down this road, you begin to notice that your walking is becoming difficult. Your joints feel as though they are stiffening, and your feet are sensitive to the roughness of the road surface. Every step you take becomes harder until you feel that you're wading painfully through a swamp, struggling to make progress.

As you continue to struggle along this route, you might choose to review some of the things that happened on your journey that brought you to this place now.

Have you found comfort in delicious food and drink like chips, chocolate, and maybe beer or wine? Everyone enjoys these little treats in life, however you are clever enough to know that it can be so easy to over-indulge, to consume more than you actually want, and more than you need to simply enjoy their simple pleasures.

Maybe you let your work or your responsibilities take priority over activity and exercise. It's only natural that you allow yourself to arrange your priorities according to your judgement about their importance. And you also understand, in this deeply relaxed state where things become clear to you, that maybe you have used these priorities as an excuse not to do something more physically challenging.

Accept and absorb this knowledge, that for everything you have ever used as a belief, you could have made a different choice, and you would not be feeling as you feel here and now.

As you continue to struggle down this route you have chosen to explore, you can feel your health and your physique deteriorating, as your heart needs to beat harder to pump the blood around your body, and the slower you get, the harder it becomes to move at all. You feel heavy and tired, and breathless. You begin to worry that some part of your body might fail, leaving you alone and stranded.

Now, you may ask yourself, was it worth it? Is this how you wanted your life to go? You worked all your life, maybe raised a family, and you always comforted yourself with the thought that you would reach your retirement years healthy, and ready to enjoy your leisure time. This feeling you have now is tired and weary, slow and cumbersome, is not what you planned or anticipated.

And you make a firm decision, right now, in your mind. You reject this future version of your life. You know it will not serve you, and you don't need it any more.

You stop, turn around, and start to walk back to fork in the road. And as you retrace your steps, it becomes easier and less painful, and you know that you have made the right decision, that you never want to go down this route again.

Now you find yourself back at the original fork in the road. And as you look up to your right, you see that the other road rises gently, and it's clear to you that this route may require some energy and effort on your part, to climb the gentle incline, however you're feeling eager to start, so you begin to walk steadily up the road on your right.

As you stroll comfortably up the gentle slope, you feel your whole body begin to respond to the increased effort, and it feels great. Now you know that when you feel yourself slowing down a little, you simply increase your pace to compensate, and you make good, strong confident progress.

Your legs feel powerful, like you could easily continue like this.

As you progress easily up this road, you appreciate the

warmth of the sun on your face and the gentle breeze at your back, and it feels like the most natural, comfortable place you could be.

As you walk, you're reminded of times when you felt like this before. Maybe when you were a child, running around and always active. And maybe you continued to be active as you grew up, and then somewhere your enthusiasm for exercise was absent, you temporarily lost something.

And now, feeling this way, strong and confident as you walk uphill, you know that you've found something that you thought was gone for good.

And you can allow yourself to feel satisfied now that this is the future you want for yourself.

Go inside and maybe you can identify the source of this good feeling, like a small glow somewhere in your body, and you can allow this feeling to grow in you, because this is how it feels when you commit, to be active each day of your life.

And you can feel that your health has changed, and you prefer your body like this.

You easily handle difficult situations or events that used to stress you out, because you've trained your body to suppress the chemicals that sent false signals to your brain.

And now you're smiling because you're enjoying yourself so much. Just allow yourself to smile and double the good feelings that you already have about yourself.

That's right - activity causes enjoyment - and you're really enjoying yourself. Feeling better and healthier and fitter than ever before.

And you've left that fork in the road a good distance behind you. You no longer need to return to that place, because you tried both options and this one, the healthy, active route, is the route you choose; this is the way you want your life to be in the future. Your desire to be fitter and healthier now energises you. You're eager to begin on your new future, a future where you feel good because you move, as often and as much as you can.

And you are aware, and it gives you great pride and satisfaction to acknowledge, that the decision you have made today is a lifelong change. You now possess all the personal resources you need to follow this route from today forwards. It is by far the best option for you and everyone who cares about you.

And you have many choices and options how you start to transform yourself to this active, energetic person you now decided to become.

You are in control. And as you carry this control into your daily life, you make good choices and decisions.

You prioritise activity, because you know it makes everything else in your life work better.

You know how good you're going to feel, so every day you look for opportunities to make a small effort, and add some activity to your life.

You love the feeling that comes with physical activity, and you chase that feeling whenever you get the chance.

You gain true enjoyment from knowing that you are changing your body each day, in preparation for a long and active life.

And as time passes these suggestions will grow stronger every day. Stronger by the hour, and the minute, and the second.

And while you allow the knowledge you are gaining to filter through your mind and find a permanent place where it becomes embedded in you attitude, habits, and behaviours, and you can allow my voice to fade gently away as you rest deeply now and restore yourself to your full energy, so just let go now and continue to drift deeper downwards....

<<Ends>>

Session 3 Transcript

So, first check yourself to make sure you're absolutely ready to go into trance, and when you know it's time, take a slow, deep breath in, hold it for a second, close your eyes, and release it at your own speed.

As the breath flows out of you, feel your body begin to anticipate how good it's going to feel to let yourself relax deeply as you've done before, and let your body relax, whilst you allow your breathing to find it's own, slow, steady rhythm, breathing in – and out – at exactly the correct speed for your body to take the nourishment it needs from each and every breath, and on your next breath in, I'd like to you to now open your eyes at the top of the breath, and then as you release the breath from your body, allow your eyes to close gently again. Good.

And now, as you breathe at your own speed, you feel your whole body begin to synchronise with your breathing, so that each time you breathe in you feel the life-giving air flowing through your whole body, and as you breathe out each time, you allow yourself to become even more deeply relaxed, feeling lazy and wonderful, and you know how good it will feel to go deeper so why not allow yourself to go all the way down now, as I start to count from ten down to one.

Ten – You are committed to finding a state of deep relaxation this time and every time you use hypnosis, and just this thought may be enough that you already begin to feel yourself more relaxed than a few moments before.

Nine – And so you have given yourself permission to do nothing else right now than allow the lazy, sensual feeling of releasing all the tension from your muscles and joints as you begin to settle into the journey to calmness and tranquillity

Eight – Deeper still, your body now so limp and floppy that you start to lose touch with your physical awareness, as you place your body in temporary hibernation – you won't be needing it for a little while, so allow it to rest

Seven – Move your attention to your face, and as you become aware of how your skin and tiny muscles of your face can easily be made to relax even more, and your face feels different now, and it's a wonderful, careless, lazy feeling as you completely release those muscles and just allow yourself to be

Six – Now your body and your face are totally relaxed and drifting safely, I'd like you to turn your attention back to your breathing and you can notice how this state of deep relaxation has slowed your breathing even more, and

Five – each time you breathe out, you naturally go deeper, as you've done before, and you possess knowledge about how effortlessly you can settle into this deepened state of consciousness, where you are the beneficiary of the personal power of change, and

Four – Now you begin to notice that your breathing is happening deeper in your body, lower down in your abdomen, and that kind of breathing feels good to you, and it is good, the best kind of breathing

Three – And now your body is at rest, and your breathing is happening at exactly the right speed, as you slowly drift down to that relaxed state that you've enjoyed so much so many times, and you know how good it feels

Two – As you start to notice that your descent is slowing as you reach the basement of your relaxation, and you may be curious about what will be the positive effect this time, and

One- You're there, totally relaxed, feeling wonderful, and you may now rest for a moment and settle into the gentle rhythm, aware of your regular, slow, controlled breathing, and allowing it to happen and your whole self to synchronise, and take a moment of silence to appreciate how you are right now...

<<Pause>>

Good, that's right.

Now that you have once more achieved this state of deep relaxation, listening only to the sound of my voice, and relaxing in rhythm with your breathing, you may begin to feel curious about what you will learn this time.

Before we get onto that, you have the opportunity to reflect on the progress you've made, and how that makes you feel. You have moved a long way from where you started, and the skills and techniques that you now possess may be some of the most useful things you'll learn in your life.

Perhaps you can begin to feel, somewhere deep inside, a tiny glow of satisfaction because you are now thinking and acting differently,

The Work

And now, combining all the knowledge you now possess, and the complete understanding and commitment that your new, motivated lifestyle is one of the most important decisions you ever made. In fact, it may be the most important decision, because its already clear to you that it's having a wonderful, refreshing effect on how you feel each day, both mentally and physically.

And you may even feel that making this change you have made is easier than you perhaps thought it would be, and maybe you sometimes wish that you made the change earlier, but that doesn't matter now, because you have made the change, and now you can use that to push yourself just a little more each day.

And even though you feel that it hasn't been difficult to make the change, its fair for us to agree that it isn't always easy to motivate yourself each day, even though you know that it's what you really want to do. Sometimes you may find yourself making a little excuse to delay something, maybe put it off until tomorrow, even though you know that you'll feel bad for the rest of the day.

That's OK to feel that way. It happens to everyone. Many people, in all walks of life, experience what you are experiencing, and many of them use a particular technique in order to overcome their inertia and move into their activities, and I'd like to show you how to do that now.

I'd like you to call on your powerful imagination now, and I'd like you to imagine you're preparing to run a sprint. Maybe you've run a race like this before, or maybe not, it doesn't matter, because I'm sure you've watched the Olympics on TV, so just allow your imagination to form an impression of yourself, in a stadium or just a school track, preparing to run.

You're already warmed up and you're waiting to be called to your marks.

See what you see, hear what you hear, feel what you feel.

Maybe you feel anticipation, excitement, or even nervousness about this race you're going to run. It must be important to you, because you've been training, but you have some tiny, nagging doubts about whether you're ready, whether you're capable of winning, whether you can stay the course to the finishing line.

And as you prepare yourself, you recall races like this that you've run before, even races you've won in the past, so you can focus on those races you ran before, and how good you felt when you won, or gave a good performance. All of the effort you put in comes back in a big rush at the end of the race.

But your nervousness grows; maybe you can feel it getting stronger somewhere in your body now, so try to locate that feeling and understand where it's coming from, and how it's affecting you.

If you allow that reluctance you are feeling now to grow too much, you might change your mind, and withdraw from the race.

Sure, that would be embarrassing, but at least you wouldn't have to risk failing. Because failing to you would be even more embarrassing than not starting in the first place.

Now you can experience the indecision for yourself. Stepping back is easy, but stepping forward is harder.

Now, holding those thoughts and feelings where they are right now, imagine you're looking down the track ahead of you, and focus on the finishing tape, which becomes clearer as you focus your attention. Crossing that tape will allow you to feel that rewarding feeling of accomplishment once again, as you have so many times before, and all you have to do is get there.

Now shift your attention to the ground directly in front of you, about a meter ahead. In your mind, draw a line across the ground, a white line, from left to right, a meter in front of you on the ground. Please do that now.

Now this line is very special. This line is called your line of commitment, and it's always there, every day, even though sometimes you forget to see it.

Your line of commitment is special because it only works one way. You can step over it from where you ar now, but you cannot step back from the other side; it simply won't allow you to step backwards.

On this side of your line of commitment, you are at rest. It might be relaxation, which you've earned and deserved, or it might be time when you're preparing, like warming up for this race you're preparing to run. While you're on this side of the line, you're stationary, not moving forwards or backwards.

You're getting ready.

Now, in a moment, but not just yet, you're going to step over the line, and when you do, you'll be in motion. Everything that happens to you after you take that step, everything you do to get yourself to the finish, from the way you set yourself in your starting blocks, to how you listen for the crack of the starter's pistol, throughout the race itself, when to push, when to cruise a little, is planned, because you've been preparing well and this is not your first race.

Go inside now and gather your energy and all the resources you need, and when you're sure that you've prepared yourself, take a longer breath than usual, and as you exhale it, step forward in your imagination, and cross your line of commitment.

And feel the change as you move from static to active, sense the forward motion, and notice how any doubts or misgivings you had are gone now, as you focus on moving forwards, making progress towards the finishing line, that goal you set for yourself, and where you know the good feelings of satisfaction and achievement will wait for you.

<<Pause>>

And you can now relax again, as you have proved your ability to discipline yourself in small and simple ways, and now you have your line of commitment, which you can create for yourself, any time you are facing tasks and challenges. Once you cross the line, you are active, and moving towards the finishing line.

And as you combine all of your skills and knowledge together, every day you feel stronger and more motivated than the day before, you have integrated your motivation as a permanent habit and behaviour.

You no longer have any need or desire to avoid or delay any activity.

Each day you actively seek out every opportunity to make progress, however small, because you know that each step forward takes you nearer to your life's goals.

You are easily able to push aside obstacles and excuses, and prioritise progress each day, because you have experienced the positive benefits your new habits bring to your life and those around you.

And I'm sure you'd agree with me that the new habits you've acquired are far more valuable than the old, unhelpful habits you have left behind, because you have now eliminated all trace of that, and you will never permit it to come back or yourself to behave in that old, out-dated way, because there is no need.

And I'd like to offer you generous portions of praise, and you can congratulate yourself on a job well done, and the changes you have made here today will stay with you from this day forwards, for the benefit of your whole life.

Good, very well done. Allow yourself to feel that pride for a few moments more.

<<Pause>>

Emerge

In a moment I'm going to count from ONE up to THREE. At the count of three your eyes are going to open, become fully alert, totally refreshed. Any sleepiness that you might have had, any dullness of mind is going to dissolve and disappear, and you're going to feel bright eyed and full of energy. You'll be fully alert and wonderful and marvellous in every way.

ONE, slowly easily and gently feel yourself coming back up to your full awareness,

At the count of TWO you're still relaxed and calm but notice that your eyes under your eyelids feel as if they're clearing, kind of like they're being bathed in a sparkling cool mountain stream, you feel GREAT.

On the next count those eyes are going to open, totally alert, fully refreshed, just feeling excited, wonderful, in every way, and every time you go into hypnosis you can let yourself go deeper than the time before because you know that just feels good.

All right, get ready, and on count of THREE open those eyes and notice how good you feel.

∼

17

PROGRAM DEBRIEF

CONGRATULATIONS! You've now completed the *Active Energy Now* program.

The new things you've learned are now firmly embedded in your subconscious, and the more you call on them, the more automatic they will become.

The more you practice, the more readily you'll be able to spin up the good feelings that go with your new active energy mindset.

You're all set, you understand the benefits.

You have the knowledge.

I wish you health and good fortune in whatever you choose to do with it.

18
OTHER RICK SMITH PROGRAMS & BOOKS

IF YOU'VE ENJOYED *Active Energy Now* here are some other programs which might interest you:

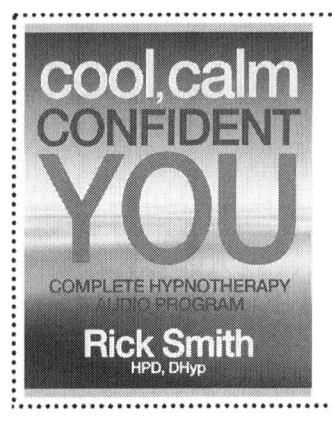

∽

COOL, CALM, CONFIDENT YOU
Complete Hypnosis Program

- 3 Full-Length Hypnosis Sessions
- 125+ Page Kindle Book
- Free Downloadable Recordings
- Includes Hypnosis Training Course

amazon kindle

What's Holding You Back?

• Maybe you're struggling with social situations? Wanting to start new friendships, but wary of putting yourself out there.

• Perhaps you want to be more confident in your work life? You've seen how more assertive people progress and succeed, and you'd like to be able to do that for yourself.

• Or are you facing presentation or performance anxiety? You have a great story to tell, but you're held back, anxious about the things that could go wrong, and ignoring the - more likely - outcome that everything goes right?

Is Shyness Stopping You Living The Life You Want?

Many people suffer all their lives, and never act. Their philosophy? If you never try, you'll never fail.

But if you never take a risk, you'll never feel the elation of a well-earned reward.

Let's Make A Change!

In **Cool, Calm, Confident You**, you'll be re-discovering strengths you've unwittingly suppressed or buried, and learning how to put them together and make them work for you.

These hypnosis tools will empower you to modify your emotional responses and remove your unnecessary obstructions to living a fuller, more confident life.

Once you've understood the rewards, you'll be highly motivated to learn and practice the methods of obtaining them.

By the time you complete the three sessions, repeating them as necessary, you'll have acquired all the tools and techniques you need to face any situation with calmness, and confidence in your ability to deal with any challenge.

Learn more on Amazon.com

Learn more on Amazon.co.uk

Or search for **rick smith hypnosis** on the Amazon bookstore.

∽

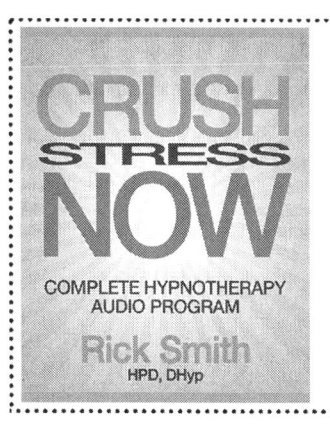

CRUSH STRESS NOW
Complete Hypnosis Program

- 3 Full-Length Hypnosis Sessions
- 125+ Page Kindle Book
- Free Downloadable Recordings
- Includes Hypnosis Training Course

amazon kindle

Stress - Take Control and Crush It, Now.

You know what it's like. That old familiar feeling starts to trouble you; it grows and mutates, sucking your energy, attention, and logical thought into a ball of aching tension, clouding your judgment and influencing your actions.

It starts in your head, but it invades your whole body, and you hate it.

Time for action...

You're Not Alone - You Can Fix Yourself

Chronic or ongoing stress can wreak havoc on your body, significantly raising your risk of serious illness. Scientists now consider underlying stress to be one of the top-three hidden killers.

The main culprit is *cortisol*, a naturally occurring, usually benign steroid hormone, which regulates many of your body's important functions. But when uncontrolled cortisol is allowed to flood your body, the damage is serious, and cumulative.

Once you understand what's happening, it's not that difficult to adapt your response so that the cortisol effects are suppressed, and you remain stable and grounded without losing your focus.

Using hypnosis, you'll learn to equalise before cortisol scores: simple techniques and routines that will enable you to remain cool and calm in the face of your challenges and navigate yourself - and those around you - through those difficult times.

By the time you complete the three sessions, repeating them as necessary, you'll have acquired all the tools and techniques you need to face any situation with calmness, and confidence in your ability to deal with any challenge.

And you'll feel a whole lot better than you do right now!

Learn more on Amazon.com

Learn more on Amazon.co.uk

Or search for **rick smith hypnosis** on the Amazon bookstore.

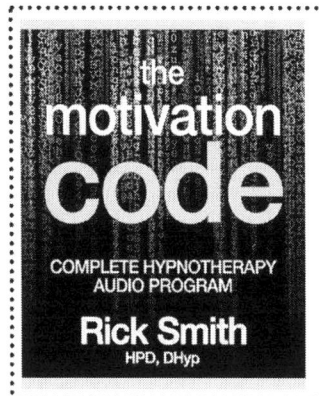

THE MOTIVATION CODE
Complete Hypnosis Program

- 3 Full-Length Hypnosis Sessions
- 125+ Page Kindle Book
- Free Downloadable Recordings
- Includes Hypnosis Training Course

amazon kindle

So, What's Holding You Back?

Whatever happened to your easy life? These days, there's so much to do. It saps your energy and your focus. Some days you just can't be bothered…

Need A Little Help to Get Moving?

Your *logical* brain knows what you need to do, and when and how to do it. But your *emotional* brain is pulling you backwards, acting like a hacker, sending you false code -

- *"Don't start that task because we might fail, and we know how that feels!"*

- *"It's so cosy here on the sofa, we can paint the fence some other time!"*

- *"We don't need a promotion, who wants to hustle that hard?"*

So you languish in your comfort zone, fooling yourself that this is the life you want, when you're actually feeling guilty, embarrassed, or ashamed because you know it's not the life you really need.

When you're demotivated like this, life can be pretty joyless.

You can be better.

Here Comes the Fix…

Your situation is your emotional *bad code*, causing you to behave sub-optimally, and it's holding you back from achieving your potential.

In the three sessions of *The Motivation Code*, we'll hunt down that broken code, and replace it with new, effective code that will fire your positive, energetic "Let's Get This Done" response instead of your old "Let's Not Bother Today" submission.

Learn more on Amazon.com

Learn more on Amazon.co.uk

Or search for **rick smith hypnosis** on the Amazon bookstore.

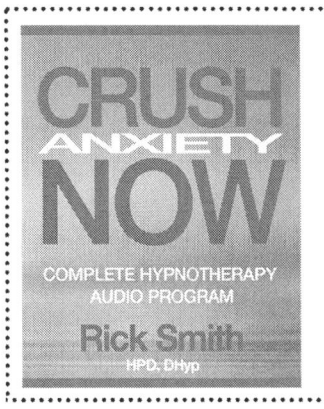

∼

CRUSH ANXIETY NOW
Complete Book & Audio Program

- 3 Full-Length Hypnosis Sessions
- 125+ Page Kindle Book
- Free Downloadable Recordings
- Includes Hypnosis Training Course

amazon kindle

Anxiety - you feel it rising, so take control and crush it, now.

You know what it's like. That old familiar feeling starts to trouble you; it grows and mutates, sucking your energy, attention, and logical thought into a ball of aching tension, clouding your judgment and influencing your actions. You hate it, and it never helps. Whatever you've tried hasn't worked, so you're looking for something different.

You're not alone - you can fix yourself

Anxiety comes in many forms, but it's usually caused by fear of something that you think is about to happen, and the way that it's going to make you feel. Your imagination perceives an impending threat and fires off a salvo of chemicals into your brain and bloodstream to alert you. Many people suffer all their lives, and never acknowledge that they need help to get on top of the condition.

Yet, once you understand what's happening, it's not that difficult to adapt your response so that the effects of these chemicals are suppressed, and you get back to normal quickly without losing your focus. Using hypnosis, you'll learn to separate your thoughts and feelings when anxiety approaches, and to focus on the outcome, not the process. You'll be able to remain cool and calm in the face of your challenges, and navigate yourself, and those around you, through those difficult situations.

By the time you complete the three sessions, repeating them as necessary, you'll have acquired all the tools and techniques you need to face any situation with calmness, and confidence in your ability to deal with any challenge.

And you'll feel a whole lot better than you do right now!

Learn more on Amazon.com

Learn more on Amazon.co.uk & eu

Or search for **rick smith hypnosis** on the Amazon bookstore.

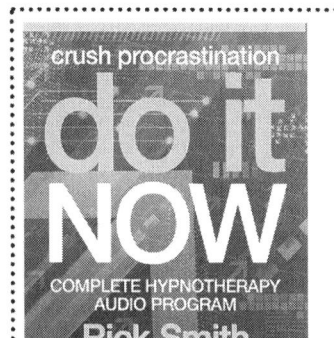

∼

DO IT NOW
Crush Procrastination

- 3 Full-Length Hypnosis Sessions
- 125+ Page Kindle Book
- Free Downloadable Recordings
- Includes Hypnosis Training Course

amazon kindle

WHY ARE You Still Putting Things Off?

Procrastination - You hate it, and it never helps. How come other people seem to get things done? You know what it's like. You've things to do but you're finding every possible reason to avoid getting started.

Why does it always have to be this way?

You're Not Alone

Many people suffer all their lives, and never acknowledge

that they need help to get on top of the bad habits and anxiety that comes with putting things off.

• Maybe you're a perfectionist? You don't want to start something because you're fearful of your ability to complete it to your own high standards, even though you may have done it – successfully - many times before.

• Or perhaps you feel inadequate or unworthy? You think – usually wrongly – that you're going to fail, so you'd rather not take the risk. Even though you know this is an illogical mind-set.

• Or is it simply that you hate the things you have to do, so you find any reason to avoid doing them? Until you absolutely have to!

You feel trapped, a hostage to procrastination.

It Doesn't Have To Be This Way

In these hypnosis sessions, we'll approach the challenge from all sides. Each recording is progressive: you'll learn and practice something and then carry that skill forwards to the next session.

By the time you complete the three sessions, you'll have mastered the capability to remain fully focused and highly motivated in every situation, knowing full well that the rewards of powering ahead are many times greater than those of holding back.

Learn more on Amazon.com

Learn more on Amazon.co.uk & .eu

Or search for **rick smith hypnosis** on the Amazon bookstore.

∼

ricksmithhypnosis.com

AFTERWORD

The Scripts Used in this Book

The recordings we used in this program can be streamed or downloaded free once you register at

http://bit.ly/AMZEnergy

If you encounter any issues obtaining the recordings, please e-mail me and I'll fix it for you.

rick@ricksmithhypnosis.com

If you enjoy the book and you find something worthwhile in the system, please take a moment to post a Review on Amazon.

However you decide to use your new skills, above all - *enjoy the journey!*

Rick Smith

Printed in Great Britain
by Amazon